An Introductory Guide to

Massage

Louise Tucker

General Editor Jane Foulston

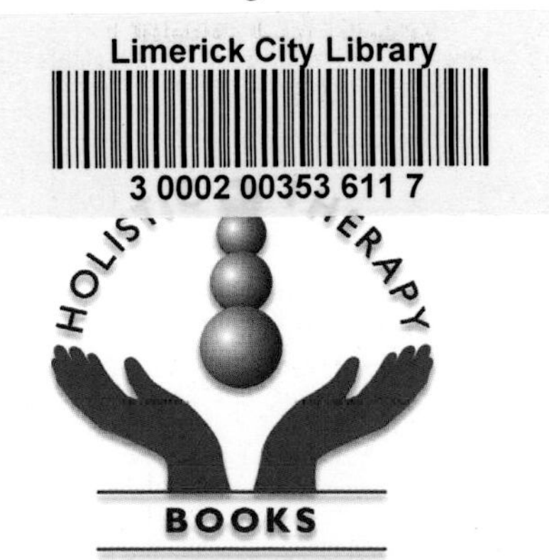

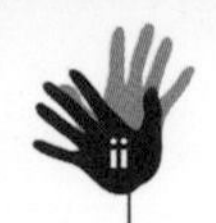

Published by Holistic Therapy Books
An imprint of Ruben Publishing Ltd.
P.O. Box 270
Cambridge
CB1 2XE

First published November 2001.
Third impression September 2004.

ISBN 1-903348-03-X.

Set in 10/13 Legacy.

Printed by Scotprint, Haddington.

Prepared for the publishers by The Write Idea, Cambridge.

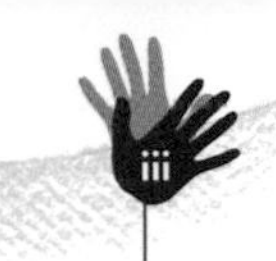

Contents

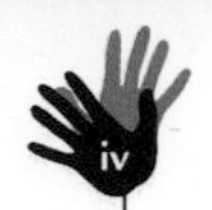

Acknowledgements

The publishers would like to thank the following for their invaluable assistance in the preparation of this book:

Heather Angel for some of the photographic images used in this book
Clare Keating-Bowman BA Hons Photography
Cariad Academy Use of premises, models and equipment

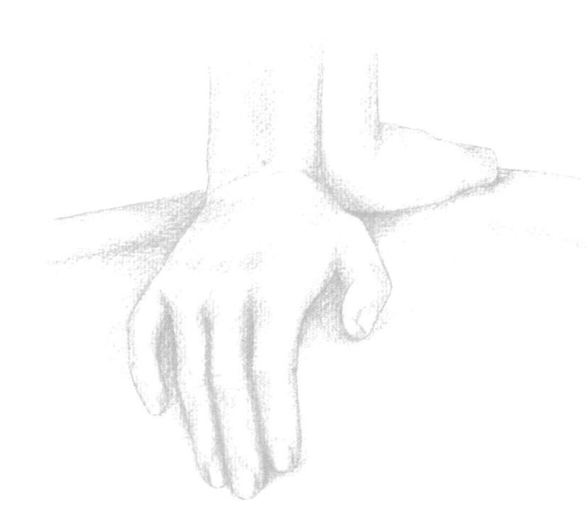

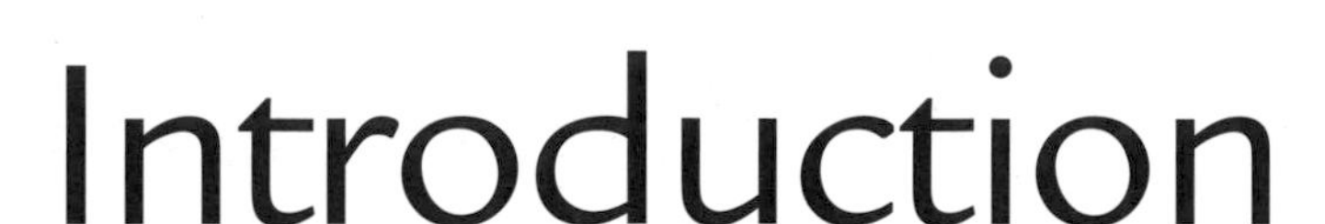

Introduction

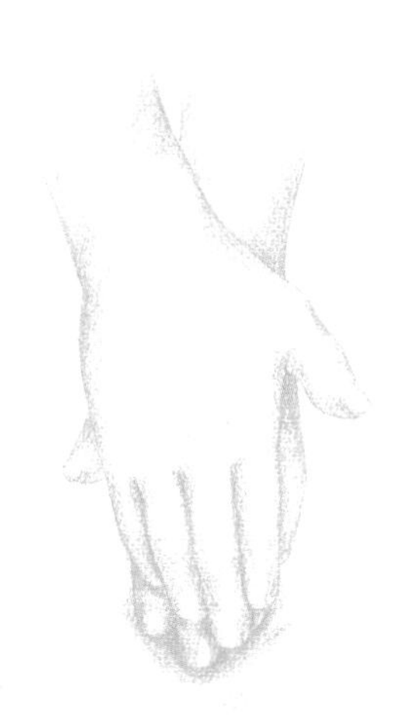

An Introductory Guide to Massage is aimed at all those starting a career in the holistic therapy of massage. Covering all the required information for carrying out a treatment, including basic anatomy, techniques and benefits, it also provides an introduction to different types of massage, such as lymphatic drainage and Indian head. It is intended for use as a textbook, as part of an accredited course, and should not be considered a substitute for professional experience and qualifications.

Author

Louise Tucker

Louise Tucker is a freelance writer. She has written several books including *An Introductory Guide to Anatomy and Physiology, An Introductory Guide to Reflexology* and *An Introductory Guide to Aromatherapy*.

General editor

Jane Foulston

Jane Foulston has had a long career as a lecturer in anatomy and physiology for beauty and complementary therapy in private and FE colleges as well as setting up a therapy school in Japan. She also has 15 years' experience as an external examiner for professional vocational qualifications. She lectured at the West of England College, East Berkshire College, Moreley College and Bridgewater College and her students have become practitioners in beauty therapy and complementary therapy and in a variety of sports therapies. She is currently Director of the International Therapy Examination Council.

Contributing editors

Marguerite Wynne

Marguerite Wynne began her career in one of London's foremost beauty salons and went on to teach in The College of Beauty Therapy in the West End. Subsequently, she owned her own clinic and school in Buckinghamshire, specialising in Complementary Therapies. She has been a Chief Examiner for ITEC since 1985 during which time she has spent three years based in the Far East.

Jill Wilshaw

Jill Wilshaw qualified in Beauty Therapy in 1980. Initially she worked in a top London Slimming Clinic before opening up her own highly successful home visiting practice in and around Harrogate. During this time she started her own private school teaching mainly Anatomy, Physiology and Massage. After relocating to Aberdeen she lectured in many subjects relating to Beauty, Complementary and Sports Therapies at Aberdeen College. She is Chief Examiner for ITEC in both practical and theory.

Note for lecturers and students

This book has been produced primarily for use by students following the ITEC massage syllabus. It has been reviewed and its content approved by ITEC for this purpose. As the publishers, we are aware, however, that there are a number of differing, and sometimes even conflicting, views on how the subject should be taught, the depth of subject matter which should be covered, and the manner in which it should be explained.

Whilst we welcome its use by anyone teaching massage therapy, we would urge lecturers and students alike to bear in mind that no text book can be all things to all people. If, as a practising therapist or lecturer, you would like to submit comments on the book which may enable us to improve future editions, they will be warmly received. We regret, however, that we are unable to enter into a discussion with regard to the accuracy or appropriacy of our interpretation.

Andy Wilson
Editorial Director

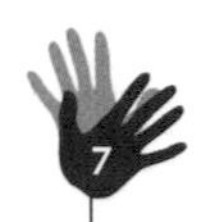

1 The history of massage and its use

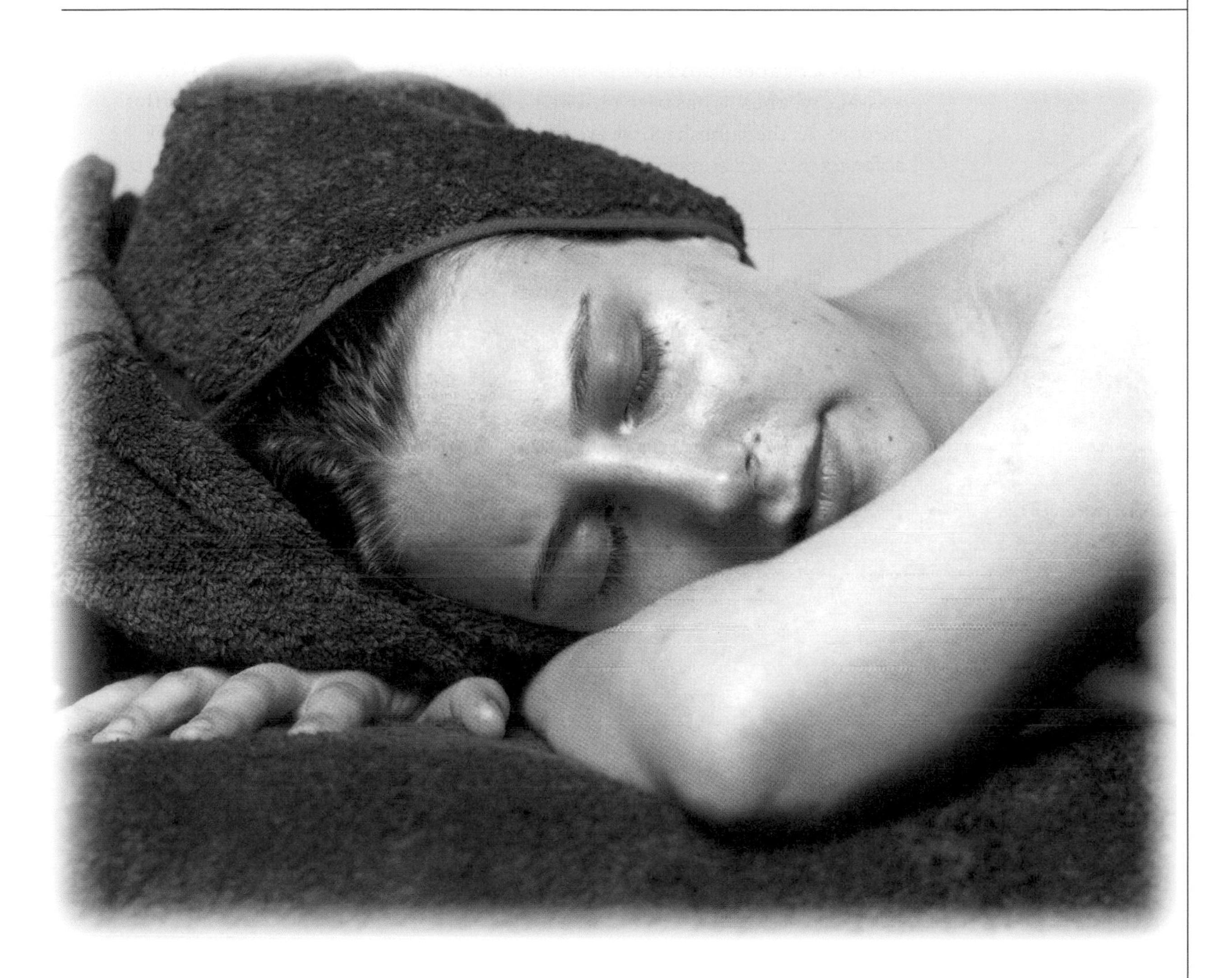

In Brief

Massage is a form of tissue manipulation which has developed over thousands of years. From ancient China to present-day Europe it has been used for the promotion and restoration of health.

Learning objectives

The target knowledge of this chapter is:
- **the history and origins of massage.**

What is massage?

Massage is the use of hands, or mechanical means, to manipulate the soft tissues of the body, particularly muscles. It can be used for relaxation, stimulation or rehabilitation of the whole body or part of it. It promotes suppleness of the muscles, improves circulation and reduces stress.

What are its main benefits and effects?

Massage is:

- *soothing:* touch is known to be soothing and comforting and massage uses touch to soothe and relax the body. Since 75% of disease is thought to be caused by stress, massage, which reduces stress, may well improve health.
- *stimulating:* the systems of the body are stimulated and activated by massage. It therefore encourages improved circulation, aids digestion, waste removal and neural communication, invigorates and relaxes muscles thus preventing spasm and stiffness, speeds up skin desquamation and promotes cell regeneration.
- *instinctive:* when we knock or hurt ourselves we often use our hands to rub or touch the affected place. Massage is an extension of this natural and instinctive method of soothing aches and pains.
- *comforting:* touch is natural and comforting. People of all ages use touch to gain a sense of security and well-being and consequently massage has psychological as well as physical benefits.
- *universal:* most people, from children to adults, can benefit from massage treatments.
- *safe:* massage is a non-threatening, non-invasive and natural therapy.

See Chapter 3 for more detailed information on the benefits and effects of massage.

Where does it come from?

Massage is not a technique derived from one culture but from many. People the world over have used touch as a form of communication, comfort and defence throughout history. Animals also use touch in a similar way, for example grooming their young with their tongues or beaks, licking wounds after a fight and nuzzling or nudging each other to show affection. The following section provides a brief history of massage technique and therapy.

THE ORIGINS AND HISTORY OF MASSAGE

What does 'massage' mean?

The word massage originates from many different languages. For example in Latin *massa* means 'that which forms a lump' and massage could be said to be a technique for removing the 'lumpiness' of the body, making it smooth. In Greek *massein* means 'to knead' and kneading is one of the fundamental movements used in this therapy. In French *masser* means 'to rub' and the basis of all massage is rubbing the skin and tissues. In Arabic *mass* means 'to touch or feel' which are both fundamental to massage.

The Ancients and massage

The use of massage has been recorded in China from 3000BC. The ancient Chinese called their technique 'amma', and used specific movements on particular points of the body. It was used for the promotion and restoration of health as well as for relaxation.
The Japanese also used the amma

technique with similar pressure points but they called the points *tsubo*. Shiatsu – the application of pressure to certain points of the body in order to improve circulation, neural efficiency and general health – uses similar points and is a direct descendant of this ancient Japanese massage practice.

In India massage has always been used as part of traditional, Ayurvedic, medicine. The Ayurveda (from Sanskrit, *ayur* meaning life and *veda* knowledge) is an ancient medical text about the arts of healing and of prolonging life and it still forms the basis of much medical knowledge in India today.

All of these countries, both in the past and present, are renowned for their holistic, or whole body, mind and spirit approach to medicine. Massage is still used as a holistic treatment, considering the whole person not just the symptom or condition.

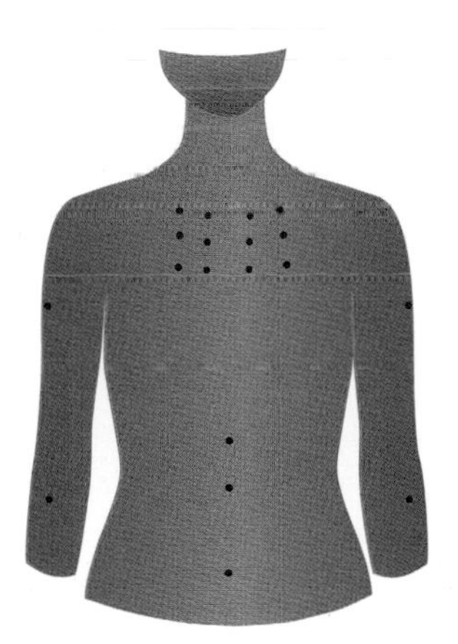

Shiatsu points on torso

The Greeks

For the Ancient Greeks massage formed part of everyday exercise and fitness. Herodicus, fifth-century physician and teacher of Hippocrates, wrote about the benefits of massage and his student Hippocrates, known as the father of medicine, believed all doctors needed to know how to use massage for healing purposes.

The Romans

At the Roman baths, which were the site of everyday social and business life for all members of society, massage was central to the whole ritual. At Turkish baths, which are the closest modern-day equivalent to Roman baths, massage is still very important. In Roman times, massage was used for treating stiff and sore muscles and joints, curing disease, strengthening the constitution and improving circulation. Gladiators were given massage before and after their bouts of fighting. A physician named Galen, who was Greek but worked for the Roman Emperor, wrote many medical books stressing the use of massage for health purposes. And, of course, Julius Caesar, the renowned Roman emperor, had massage daily.

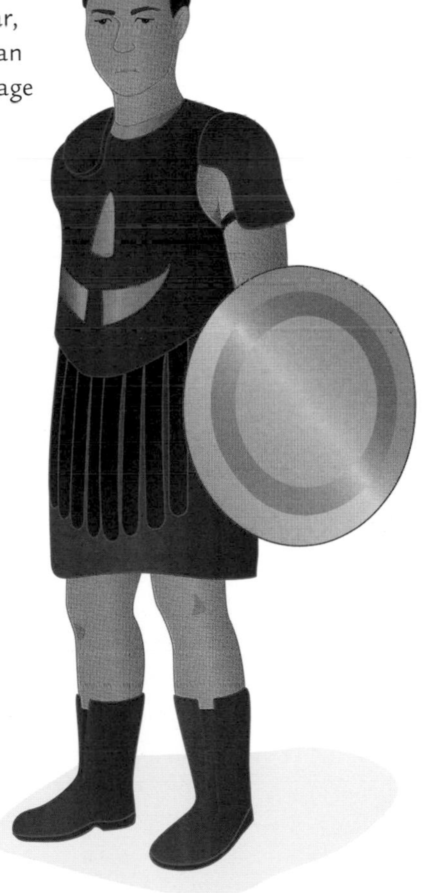

A Roman gladiator

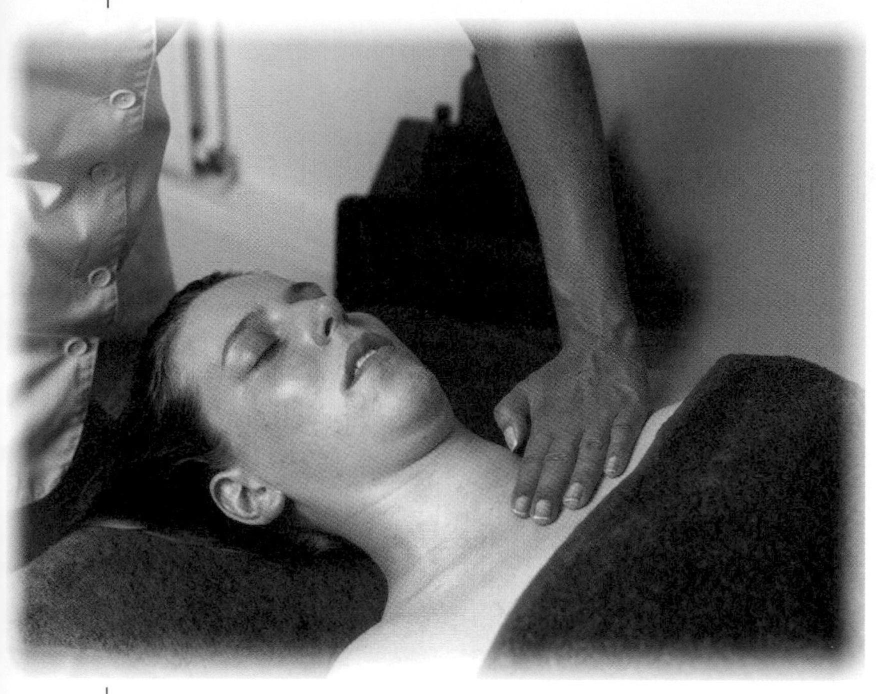

Facial massage

Modern massage

Modern massage is based on techniques developed by Per Henrik Ling (1776-1839), a physiologist and fencing master. He was from Sweden and massage is still referred to as Swedish massage because of his influence. In the eighteenth and nineteenth centuries, having studied in China, he developed a system of movements which he found helpful for improving his health and maintaining his physical condition. These movements are known as the Ling System and include techniques known as passive and active. His work was recognised first in his home country – in 1813 the Swedish government established the Royal Swedish Central Institute of Gymnastics of which Ling was named President – and subsequently around the world. In 1838 the Swedish Institute opened in London and there are now similar institutes in other countries.

Massage in the late nineteenth and early twentieth centuries

At the end of the nineteenth century massage was battling for respectability. The name was often used in relation to prostitution and therefore the therapy was not taken seriously. However, in order to combat this eight women founded The Society of Trained Masseuses in 1884. This later became the Chartered Society of Physiotherapy. Massage continued to be used extensively for medical purposes by doctors.

In the two world wars massage was used to treat nerve injury and for rehabilitation. However, around this time mechanical methods of treatment began to replace manual methods. This led to a reduction in the use of therapeutic massage and a lack of awareness of its benefits.

Massage now

Massage has, in recent years, once again become a reputable and recognised therapy, thanks to an increased awareness of and interest in complementary therapies and alternative medicine. Many systems and methods exist but Swedish massage remains the basis for most practice. It can be used alone or in combination with other treatments and is a central part of therapies such as physiotherapy, stress-management and aromatherapy.

Massage is beneficial to all body systems and is a natural and effective way to treat both physical conditions and psychological problems.

You now know the origins of massage.

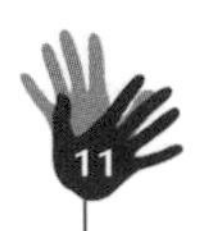

2 Anatomy for massage

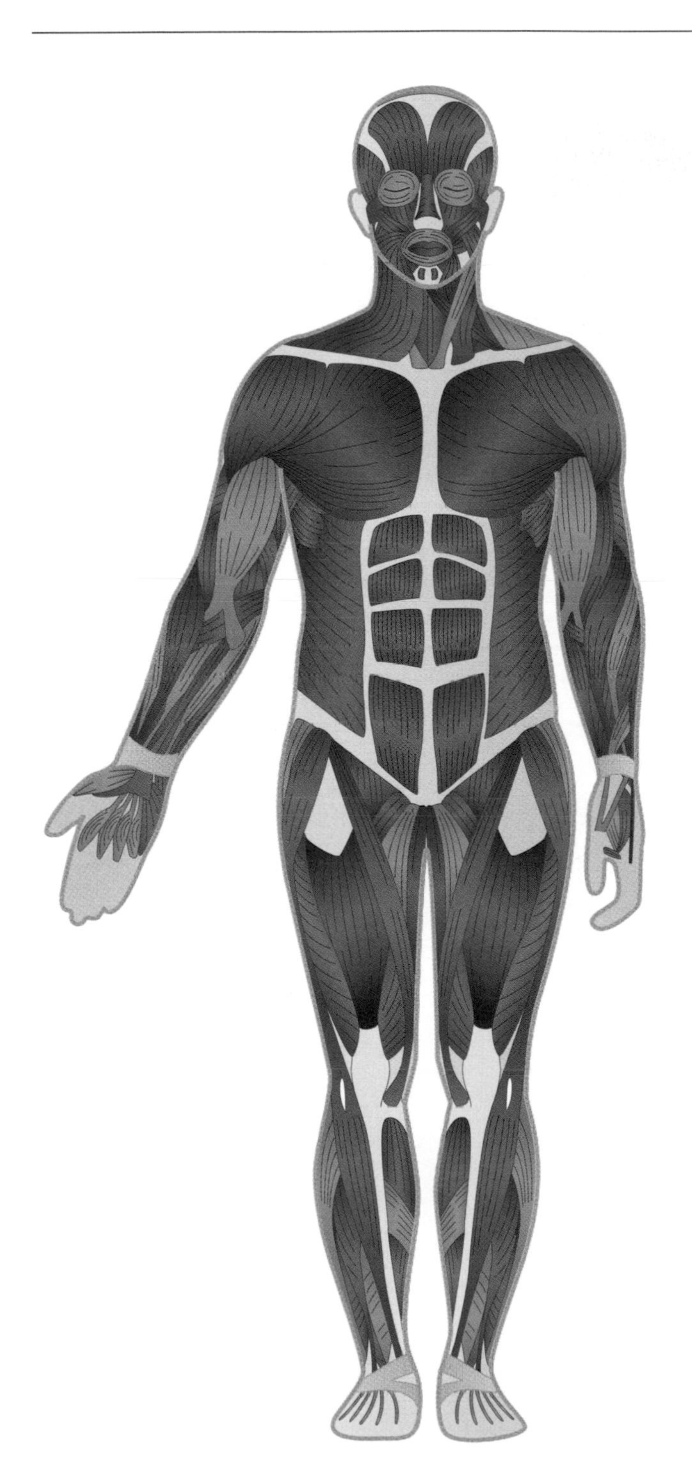

In Brief

Massage benefits the whole body, both physiologically and psychologically. However, some of the systems are more directly affected, particularly the skin, blood and lymph circulation, muscles and nerves. In order to understand how massage affects and benefits these systems it is useful to learn about their structure, their function and the diseases that affect them.

Learning objectives

The target knowledge of this chapter is:

- structure, function and diseases of the skin
- structure, function and diseases of the circulatory (vascular) system
- structure, function and diseases of the lymphatic system
- structure, function and diseases of the muscular system
- structure, function and diseases of the nervous system

THE SKIN

What is it?

The skin is the body's outer protective layer, also known as the integumentary system. It is the largest organ in the body, covering every part including the eyes, and varies in thickness. For example the skin on the soles of the feet is much thicker than the skin of the eyelids. There are two layers of skin, the epidermis and dermis or 'true skin', underneath which is the subcutaneous layer.

The epidermis is the skin that we see and is itself made up of layers of cells. The cells in the epidermis are constantly being desquamated (slowly rubbed off the body) and replaced. The dermis is the layer below the epidermis. This part of the skin contains blood, lymph and nerve vessels as well as sweat glands, sebaceous glands, hair follicles and living cells.

What does the skin do?

The skin has many functions:

- it secretes sebum, a natural moisturiser, from the sebaceous glands. Sebum lubricates the hair shafts, moisturises the skin and, combined with perspiration helps to form a barrier against bacteria called the acid mantle
- it helps regulate body temperature through vasodilation and vasoconstriction
- it waterproofs the body, although some substances can be absorbed, including certain drugs and essential oils
- it protects the body: its natural acid pH prevents bacterial invasion; melanin contained in the basal layer of the epidermis helps to protect the skin against damage from ultraviolet light

Cross-section of skin

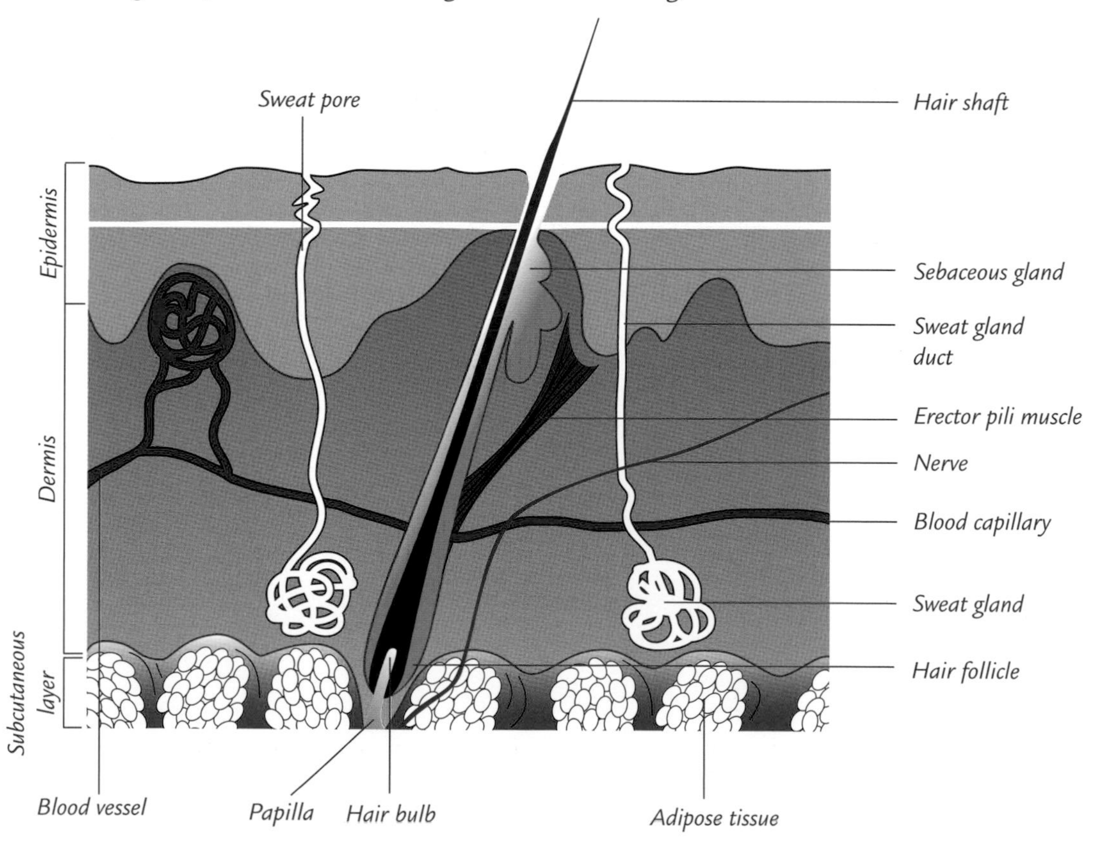

- it eliminates waste through sweating
- it is the organ of touch, acting both as an information and warning system, telling the body about pain, pressure, heat and cold as well as the comfort and pleasure of contact
- it produces vitamin D, essential for the formation and maintenance of bone
- it produces melanin, the tanning pigment which darkens the skin in order to protect it from ultraviolet radiation.

Diseases of the skin

Massage therapists are in constant contact with the skin of their clients. It is therefore very important to be able to recognise skin conditions/diseases both for their own safety and that of the client.

Congenital conditions

These conditions may be inherited and often exist from birth.

- **Eczema**

The skin develops scaly, itchy, dry patches, sometimes with points of bleeding. It is found all over the body, but especially in the crook of the elbow, behind the knees, on the face, hands and scalp. It is not contagious. Not all forms of eczema are congenital. Atopic eczema occurs in people who may have an inherited tendency to allergy. Other forms of eczema (e.g. hand eczema) may be the result of irritation.

- **Psoriasis**

A chronic inflammation of the skin which causes red patches covered with silvery scales that are constantly shed. The size of the patches varies from minute points to whole limbs, with occasional bleeding. Psoriasis affects the whole body, particularly the knees, elbows, scalp, lower back and arms. It is not contagious.

- **Dermatitis**

Allergic reaction to substances that have either been taken in or come into contact with the skin. The skin is usually red and itchy and there may be tiny raised vesicles (blisters) which can burst, forming a dry crust which can crack and cause bleeding. This could cause a secondary infection.

Bacterial conditions

- **Acne rosacea**

This is an eruption which affects the face, nose and cheeks. It has a red, flushed appearance and may be lumpy and thick with possible pustules. It can be associated with the menopause or other hormonal changes, therefore it is more common in women than men. It is aggravated by hot, spicy foods, caffeine, alcohol and changes in temperature. Not contagious.

- **Acne vulgaris**

The skin develops papules, pustules and comedones and has a shiny, sallow appearance. Acne vulgaris may be caused by hormonal imbalances, particularly in puberty, resulting in over-active sebaceous glands. The excess of sebum blocks the pores and causes infection. It mainly affects the face, back, chest and shoulders. Although not contagious, acne vulgaris is contraindicated because touching the affected area can spread the condition or burst pustules.

- **Boils**

An infection which causes inflammation around a hair follicle. Avoid touching the area during massage.

- **Folliculitis**

An infection of the sebaceous gland and hair follicle which causes inflammation and often occurs in conjunction with acne vulgaris. Avoid touching during massage. Common on buttocks, thigh, neck and armpits.

- **Impetigo**

A highly contagious infection which causes blisters which weep and develop a thick, yellow crust. Common around the nose and mouth. Contraindicated.

Viral conditions

Massage is contraindicated for these viral conditions because they are highly contagious.

- **Herpes simplex**

Herpes simplex is commonly known as a cold sore. It causes small blisters which usually occur on the mouth but can spread to other parts of the body. The blisters eventually dry up forming a crust which falls off. Contagious.

- **Herpes zoster**

This viral infection is commonly known as shingles and is the adult form of chicken pox. It is a nervous system disorder, usually affecting the spinal nerves and one side of the thorax and causes a rash of blisters with very severe itching. Highly contagious.

- **Warts**

Growths on the skin, of which there are many types. Avoid the area.

- **Verrucas**

Warts found on the feet. Avoid the area.

Fungal conditions

Fungal conditions are infections which attach themselves mainly to keratinised structures such as the skin. Massage is contraindicated for fungal conditions which are highly infectious.

- **Tinea corporis**

This is also known as ringworm and is found all over the body.

- **Tinea pedis**

This is commonly known as athlete's foot and is found on the feet.

Other

- **Allergic reactions including urticaria**

When the skin is irritated it produces histamine as a defence. This can cause watery, stinging eyes, itching, swellings, red blotchy patches and a runny nose. Urticaria (also known as nettle rash or hives) is a severe allergic reaction characterised by pinkish weals. Therapists should ensure at consultation stage that the client has no allergies that may be provoked by massage or the medium used.

- **Skin cancer**

Skin cancer is caused by excessive exposure to sunlight and contraindicated for massage because of the risk of spreading it.

- **Basal cell carcinoma**

The skin develops nodules or shallow ulcers with raised edges. It occurs on exposed parts of the skin, especially face, nose, eyelid, cheek and is the least malignant skin cancer.

- **Squamous cell carcinoma**

Squamous cells are the type of cell found on the top layer of the skin. This cancer consists of a swelling, that may resemble a wart or ulcer, that grows rapidly.

- **Malignant melanoma**

A malignant tumour of melanocytes (the cells that produce melanin). It usually develops in a previously benign mole. The mole may become larger and darker, and may itch or bleed. The tumour eventually spreads. This is the most malignant skin cancer.

You now know what the skin is, what it does and the types of diseases that affect it.

THE CIRCULATORY (VASCULAR) SYSTEM

What is it?

The circulatory system is the body's transport system, composed of the heart, blood and blood vessels. Blood carries the body's fuel and the heart is the body's engine. The heart pumps blood around the body in a system of vessels known as arteries, veins and capillaries.

Arteries carry oxygenated (arterial) blood from the heart and veins carry deoxygenated (venous) blood back to the heart. Capillaries are tiny porous vessels at the end of the arteries which distribute oxygen, nutrients and fluid and collect carbon dioxide, waste and fluid.

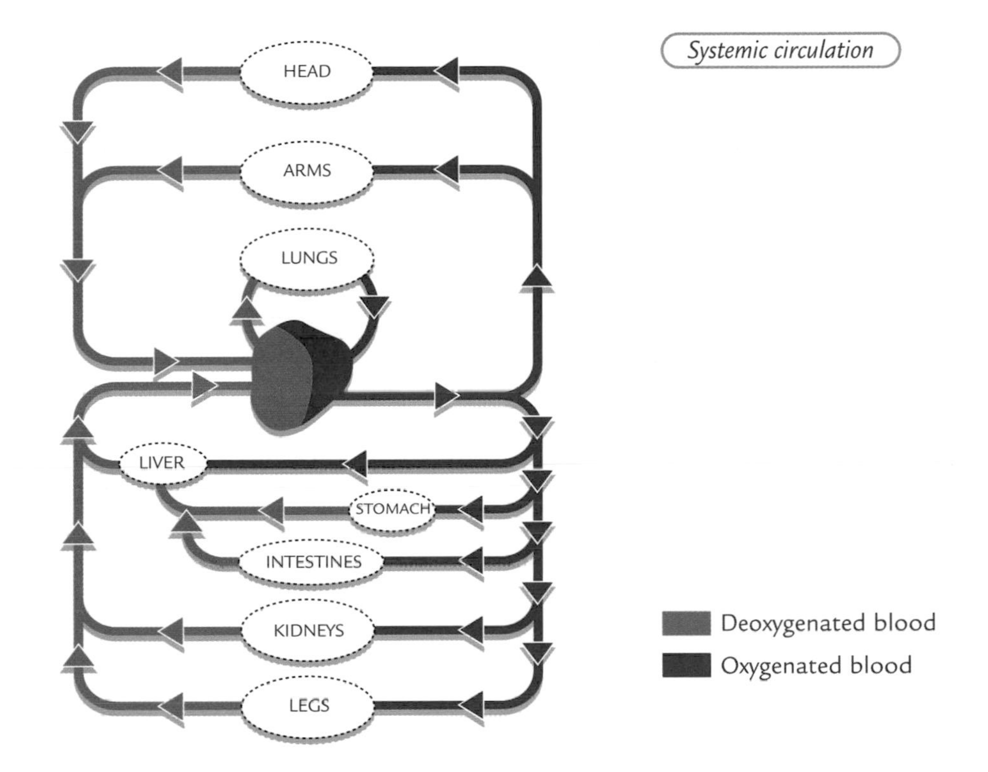

What does it do?

It pumps and transports blood, a fluid connective tissue consisting of different types of cells which is used to distribute nutrients and oxygen to the tissues, and waste and carbon dioxide from the tissues. Blood also carries hormones and contains cells that help fight infection (leucocytes). It also transports heat and therefore helps with heat regulation.

Diseases of the circulatory system

Massage stimulates the circulation so any circulatory disorders may be aggravated by it. The therapist should ensure that the client has no contra-indicated circulatory diseases at the consultation stage and contact the client's GP if in any doubt about the suitability of treatment.

Anaemia

Anaemia is a reduction in the blood's ability to carry oxygen, caused either by a decrease in red blood cells, or the haemoglobin they carry, or both. It may be caused by extensive loss of blood, lack of iron in the diet, the failure of bone marrow to produce the normal level of cells or it may be inherited.

Arteriosclerosis
A degenerative disease of the arteries, in which the walls of the vessels harden and lose elasticity. The loss of elasticity causes an increase in blood pressure. This condition mainly affects the elderly.

Atherosclerosis
A build-up of fats, including cholesterol, inside the arteries which causes a narrowing of the artery passage, hardening of the vessel walls and a loss of elasticity.

Haemophilia
The blood's inability to clot. This is an inherited disease which affects mainly men but which can be carried by women.

Haemorrhoids
Also known as piles, these are enlarged veins in the rectum or anus which may collapse or contain blood clots.

Heart conditions
Any client with a history of heart disease, angina or heart attacks should have treatment approved by a GP.

Hepatitis A B C
Inflammations of the liver, caused by viruses, toxic substances or immunological abnormalities. Type A is spread by fecally contaminated food. Types B and C are transmitted by infected body fluids including blood. Contagious.

High blood pressure
High blood pressure (hypertension) is blood pressure that consistently remains above the normal level. It is caused by many different factors including stress, poor diet, smoking and obesity. Stimulating massage may aggravate this condition because it invigorates the circulation. If the client suffers from hypertension, the therapist will need to check with the GP that massage is safe as the client may be taking medication for their condition that might result in fluctuations in blood pressure.

High cholesterol
High cholesterol is an excessive build-up of a fatty substance called cholesterol, which can cause a reduction in arterial capacity (atherosclerosis – see previous page) and thus high blood pressure.

Leukaemia
Leukaemia is a cancer of the blood, caused by over-production of white blood cells.

Low blood pressure
Low blood pressure (hypotension) is blood pressure that consistently remains below the normal level. It is not usually contraindicated for massage unless severe, in which case the GP should be consulted and then, if safe, the therapist should carry out a gentle massage as even with gentle massage blood pressure will drop once the parasympathetic nervous system is stimulated.

Phlebitis
Inflammation of a vein. Thrombophlebitis is the inflammation of a vein where a blood clot has formed.

Stress
Stress can be defined as any factor which affects mental or physical health. When a person is stressed, the heart beats faster, thus pumping blood more quickly. Excessive and unresolved stress can lead to high blood pressure, coronary thrombosis and heart attacks.

Thrombosis
A blood clot in a blood vessel. Always contraindicated because massage may move it and cause further complications.

Varicose veins

Varicose veins are caused by the collapse of valves in veins and are commonly found in the lower legs. Venous blood has to travel uphill in order to return to the heart and valves in the veins help prevent backward flow. Sometimes these valves no longer work effectively and the venous blood collects, dilating and distending the veins, creating bluish knobbly veins. Massage should only be used above and not directly on varicose veins as this may weaken them further and can be very painful for the client.

You now know what the circulatory system is, what it does and the types of diseases that affect it.

THE LYMPHATIC SYSTEM

What is it?

The lymphatic system is a secondary circulation which is intertwined with and supports the blood. It consists of lymphatic vessels, lymph nodes, lymphatic ducts and lymph.

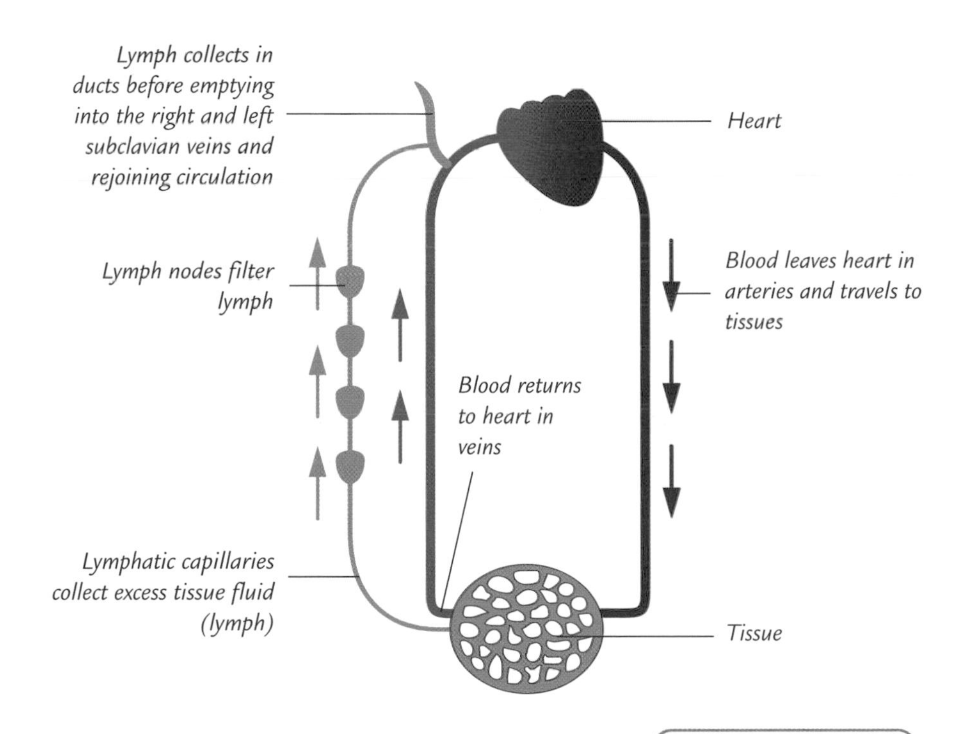

Lymph circuit (simplified)

What does it do?

The lymphatic system drains excess tissue fluid from the spaces around tissues, rather than from the tissues themselves. Excess fluid and large particles in the tissue spaces that cannot pass back through the small pores of the capillaries are collected by lymphatic capillaries. They transport this fluid, known as lymph, to lymph vessels and then to lymph nodes which filter it to remove any waste, toxins or bacteria. The lymphatic system also protects against infection and disease by producing antibodies and white blood cells, known as lymphocytes, in lymph nodes. These protective cells are added to the lymph before it is returned to the circulation.

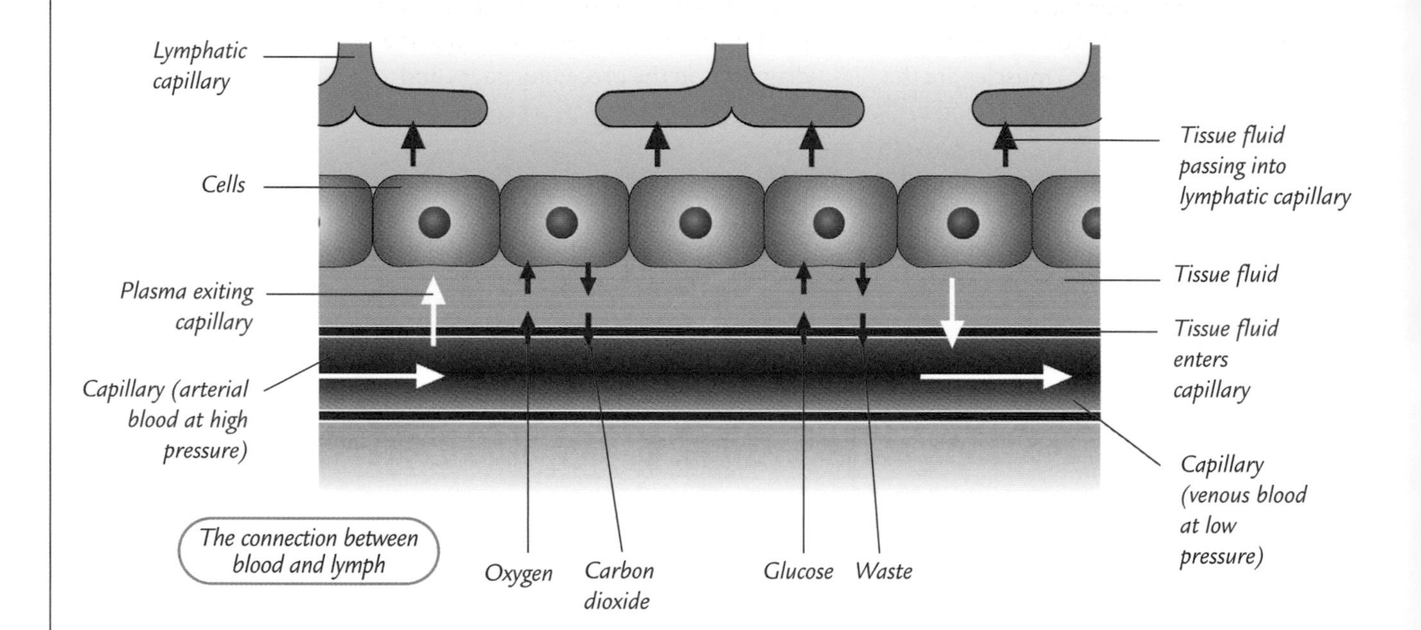

The connection between blood and lymph

Diseases and disorders of the lymphatic system

Massage improves lymphatic circulation. Any fever or infection is contraindicated not only because it is unsafe for the therapist but also because it may be spread by the treatment.

Lymphoedema

Lymphoedema is a form of swelling caused by a malfunction of the lymphatic system. It is caused by poor drainage either because the lymph vessels have been damaged or the lymph has become trapped. As with varicose veins poor lymph drainage can start a cycle: once lymph gets trapped and collects it then sits in the vessel stretching and distending it which causes poor drainage. Lymphoedema usually affects the arms or legs. Massage, particularly lymphatic drainage massage, can be very beneficial. See Chapter 8 for more details.

Hodgkin's disease

Cancer of the lymphoid tissue. The lymphatic nodes swell painlessly, either in one area or several. Other symptoms include weight loss, weakness, itchiness, fever, anaemia and lowered immunity. Contraindicated.

You now know what the lymphatic system is, what it does and the types of diseases that affect it.

THE MUSCULAR SYSTEM

What is the muscular system?

The muscular system consists of muscles and their attachments, known as tendons and fascia, which connect the muscles to bones and joints. There are three types of muscle, cardiac, involuntary and voluntary. Cardiac muscle is only found in the heart and works to pump blood around the body. Involuntary (smooth) muscles are the muscles that we do not consciously control, such as those in the walls of blood vessels. Voluntary (skeletal) muscles are the muscles that we consciously control, such as those in our arms and legs.

What does the muscular system do?

The muscular system enables movement. Muscles consist of muscle fibres and when these fibres contract the muscle changes shape and moves the part of the body to which it is attached. Muscles also stabilise the joints, help control body temperature through shivering and dilation of the capillaries and maintain postural tone. At any one time, however relaxed we might think we are, there are muscles contracting in order for us to sit, stand or lie down.

Why is it important to know about muscles for massage?

Throughout a massage, the therapist's movements are working over muscles and it is very important to know which voluntary muscles are being treated at any time, what they do (their action) and how the massage may affect them. Voluntary or skeletal muscles usually have two ends, known as the origin (part closest to the midline/body and the part which is the fixed end of the muscle and therefore hardly moves) and the insertion (part furthest away from midline and the moving end of the muscle). Muscles always work from their insertion to their origin and when massaging, movements are usually carried out in the direction of the heart, therefore from the insertion towards the origin. It is important to understand the position of the muscles as shown in the diagrams on the preceding pages and their action. The following table details the origin, insertion and action of the major muscles of the body.

Diseases of the muscular system

Massage movements directly affect the muscles and are generally beneficial for most conditions affecting them.

Atony

Lack of normal tone or tension in a muscle.

Atrophy

Caused by ndernourishmentor lack of use. The effects are wasting away, or failure to reach normal size, of bulk of muscle.

Cramp

Cramp is a sustained involuntary contraction of a muscle, perhaps caused by salt deficiency. Massage is one of the most effective ways of relieving cramp.

Fibrositis

Build-up of lactic acid inside the muscles causing inflammation of tissues, stiffness and pain. Lumbago is a form of fibrositis of the muscles in the lumbar area of the back. Torticollis, or 'wry neck' is a form of fibrositis of the sternocleidomastoid muscle in the neck which causes the head to lean to one side.

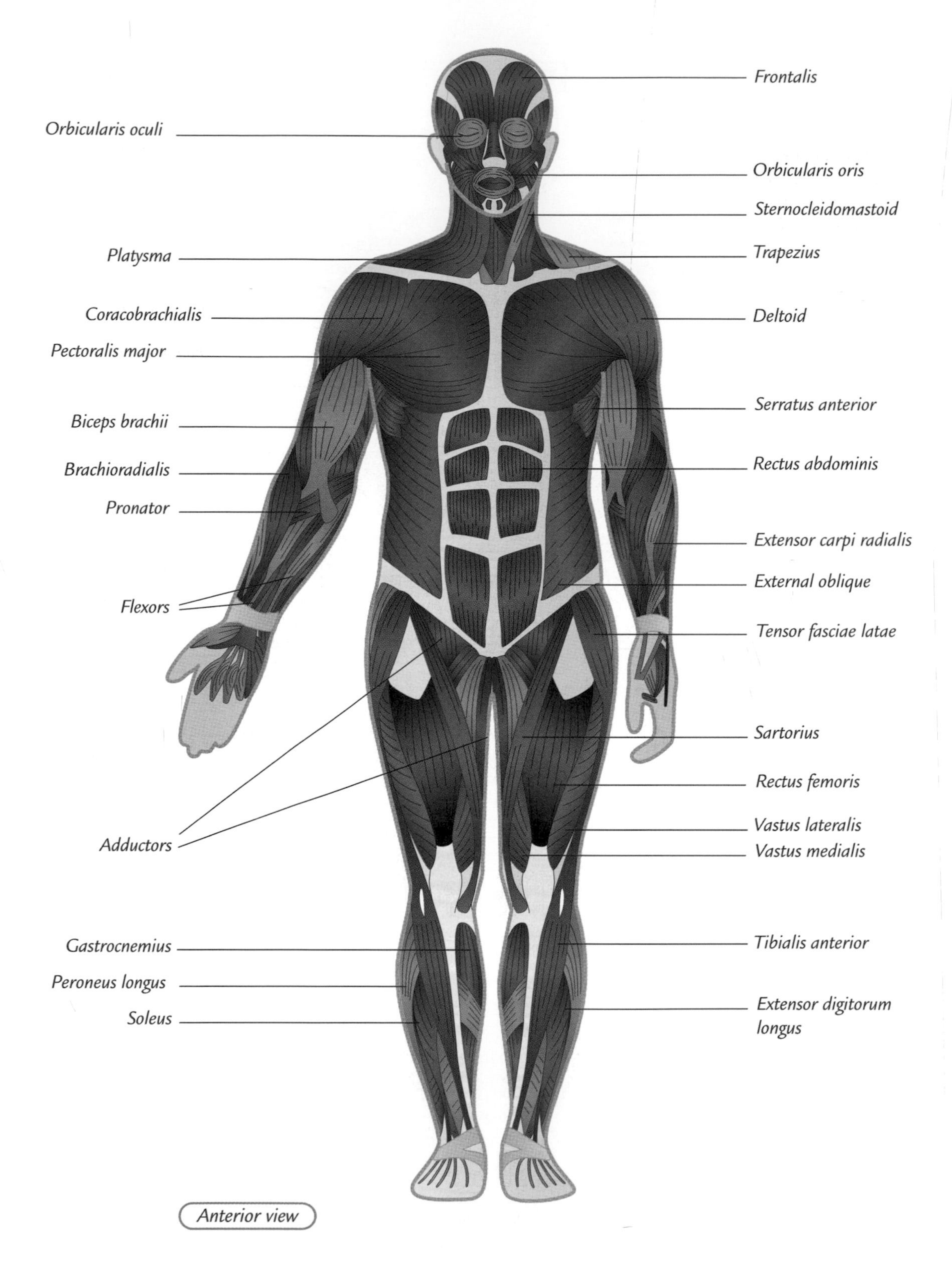

Anterior view

NB The exact position of some muscles cannot be shown as they are underneath other muscles. The positions indicated are intended as a general guide only.

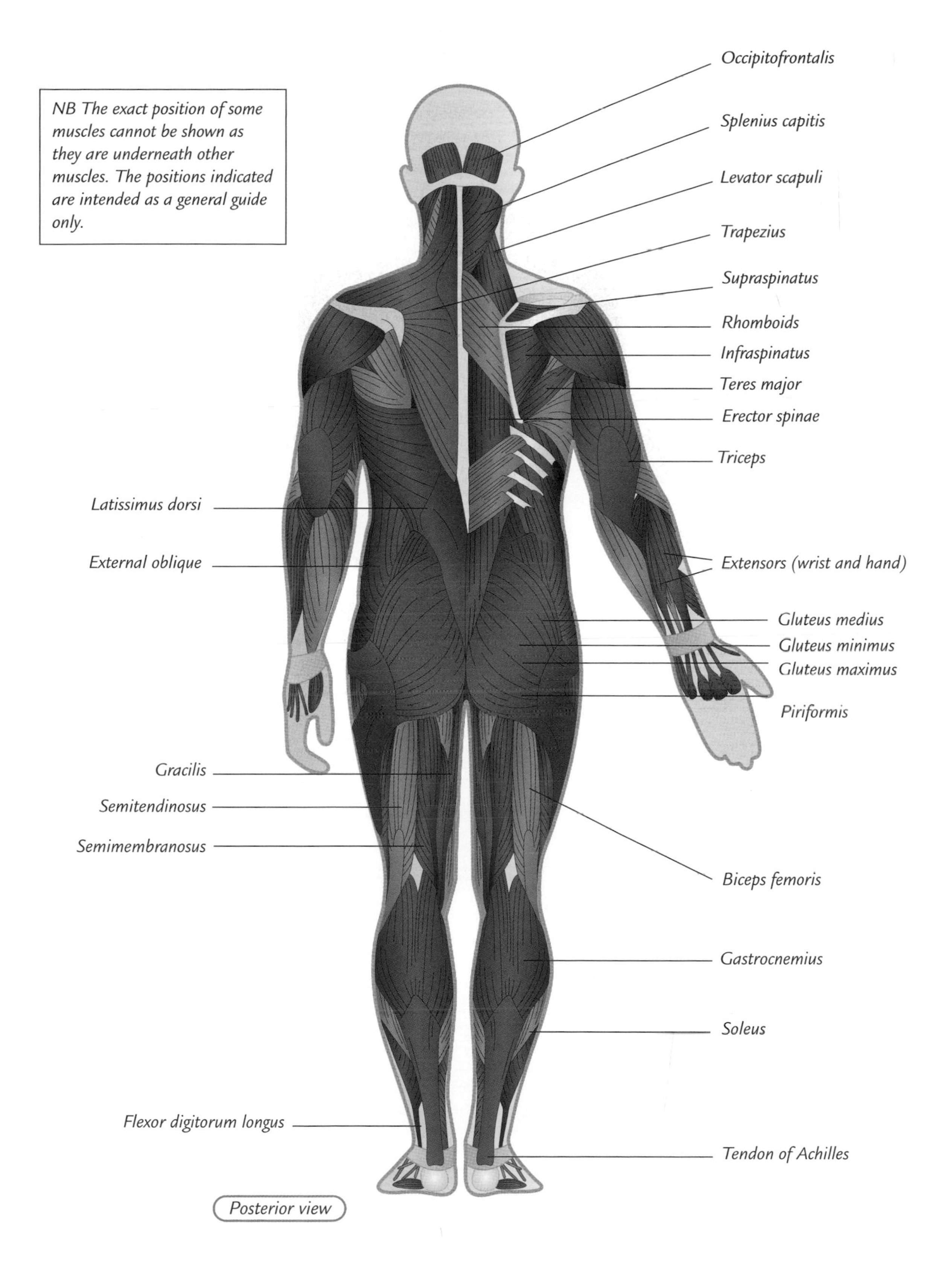

Posterior view

Muscles of the torso	Origin	Insertion	Main actions
Sternocleidomastoid	Sternum & clavicle	Mastoid process	One side only – flexes neck laterally and rotates it Both – side flexion
Scalenes	Transverse processes of 2nd to 6th cervical	Upper surfaces of ribs 1 and 2	Raises first two ribs, flexes and rotates the neck
Splenius capitis	First six thoracic vertebrae	Mastoid process and occipital bone	Extends the neck Slight rotation
Levator scapulae	Upper four cervical vertebrae	Superior medial border of scapula	Elevates shoulder, rotates scapula
Supraspinatus	Supraspinous fossa of scapula	Greater tuberosity of humerus	Abducts arm
Infraspinatus	Inferior spinous fossa of scapula	Greater tuberosity of humerus	Rotates arm outwards (laterally)
Subscapularis	Subscapular fossa of scapula	Lesser tuberosity of humerus	Rotates arm inwards
Teres minor	Axillary border of scapula	Greater tuberosity of humerus	Rotates arm outwards (laterally)
Teres major	Inferior angle of scapula	Medial lip of bicipital groove of humerus	Draws arm backwards, adducts and medially rotates it
Rhomboid major & minor	7th cervical and 1st to 5th thoracic vertebrae	Medial border of scapula	Adducts (draws towards spine) and rotates scapula downwards
Trapezius	Occipital bone, cervical and thoracic vertebrae	Clavicle and spine of scapula Acromion process	Elevates and braces shoulder, rotates scapula
Latissimus dorsi	Lower six thoracic and lumbar vertebrae Sacrum and illiac crest	Bicipital groove of humerus	Draws arm backwards, adducts and rotates it inwards
Erector spinae	Sacrum and iliac crest, ribs and lower vertebrae	Ribs, vertebrae and mastoid process,	One side only – flexes trunk laterally Both – extends trunk
Quadratus lumborum	Iliac crest	12th rib and transverse processes of upper four lumbar vertebrae	One side only – flexes trunk laterally and rotates it Both – extends trunk
Pectoralis major	Clavicle, sternum, upper six costal cartilages	Lateral lip of bicipital groove of humerus	Draws arm forwards (flexes) and adducts and rotates it inwards (medial rotation)
Pectoralis minor	3rd to 5th ribs	Coracoid process of scapula	Draws shoulder forwards and downwards
Serratus anterior	Upper nine ribs	Anterior surface of vertebral border of scapula	Draws shoulder forwards and rotates scapula
Rectus abdominus	Pubis	Ribs and sternum	Flexes the trunk
Abdominus tranversalis	Inguinal ligament, iliac crest, lumbar fascia, cartilages of lower six ribs	Conjoint tendon and linea alba through abdominal aponeurosis, pubis	Supports the viscera, compresses abdomen

Muscles of the torso (cont)	Origin	Insertion	Main actions
Internal obliques	Inguinal ligament, iliac crest and lumbar fascia	Costal cartilages of ribs 9–12 and linea alba	Lumbar flexion, side flexion and rotation
External obliques	Lower eight ribs	Iliac crest and linea alba through abdominal aponeurosis	Lumbar flexion, side flexion and rotation
Muscles of the arm			
Deltoid	Clavicle, acromion process and spine of scapula	Deltoid tuberosity of humerus	Front draws arm forwards Middle abducts the arm Back draws arm backwards
Coracobrachialis	Coracoid process of scapula	Shaft of humerus	Adducts and flexes the arm, horizontally adducts the shoulder
Biceps brachii	Long head – supra glenoid tubercle of scapula Short head – coracoid process of scapula	Tuberosity of radius	Flexes elbow, supinates forearm
Brachialis	Shaft of humerus	Coronoid process of ulna	Flexes elbow
Brachioradialis	Lateral condyloid ridge of humerus	Distal part of radius	Flexes elbow
Triceps brachii	Long head – scapula Medial head – humerus Lateral head – humerus	Olecranon process of ulna	Extends elbow
Anconeus	Lateral epicondyle of humerus	Olecranon process of ulna	Extends elbow
Pronator teres	Above medial epicondyle of humerus and coronoid process of ulna	Middle of shaft of radius	Pronates forearm and hand
Supinator	Lateral epicondyle of humerus	Lateral surface of radius	Supinates forearm and hand
Extensor digitorum	Lateral epicondyle of humerus	Metacarpals and phalanges	Extends wrist and fingers
Extensor carpi radialis brevis & longus	Lateral epicondyle of humerus	2nd and 3rd metacarpals	Extends and abducts wrist
Extensor carpi ulnaris	Lateral epicondyle of humerus	5th metacarpal	Extends wrist
Flexor carpi radialis	Medial epicondyle of humerus	2nd and 3rd metacarpals	Flexes wrist
Flexor carpi ulnaris	Medial epicondyle of humerus and ulna	5th metatcarpal, pisiform and hamate	Flexes wrist
Muscles of the leg			
Iliopsoas Psoas Iliacus	12th thoracic and all lumbar vertebrae, iliac fossa and front of sacrum	Lesser trochanter of femur	Flexes and medially rotates hip
Gluteus maximus	Posterior crest of ilium, posterior surface of sacrum and coccyx	Gluteal tuberosity of femur	Tenses fascia lata and extends hip, raises trunk after stooping

Muscles of the leg (cont)	Origin	Insertion	Main actions
Gluteus medius	Posterior surface of ilium	Greater trochanter of femur	Abducts and medially rotates femur
Gluteus minimus	Lateral surface of ilium	Greater trochanter of femur	Abducts and medially rotates femur
Piriformis	Front of sacrum	Greater trochanter of femur	Laterally rotates femur
Tensor fascia lata	Anterior iliac crest	Fascia lata	Abducts and rotates the femur
Biceps femoris	Long head – ischium Short head – linea aspera	Head of fibula and lateral condyle of tibia	Extends hip, flexes knee
Semimembranosus	Ischial tuberosity	Medial condyle of tibia	Extends hip, flexes knee
Semitendinosus	Ischial tuberosity	Below medial condyle of tibia	Extends hip, flexes knee
Rectus femoris	Above acetabulum	Through patella and patellar tendon on to tibial tuberosity	Extends knee, flexes hip
Vastus lateralis	Greater trochanter and linea aspera	Through patella and patellar tendon on to tibial tuberosity	Extends knee
Vastus intermedius	Shaft of femur	Through patella and patellar tendon on to tibial tuberosity	Extends knee
Vastus medialis	Whole length of linea alba and medial condyloid ridge	Through patella and patellar tendon on to tibial tuberosity	Extends knee
Sartorius	Anterior superior iliac spine	Below medial condyle of tibia	Flexes, abducts and rotates femur laterally, flexes knee
Gracilis	Pubis and ischium	Below medial condyle of tibia	Adducts and medially rotates femur, flexes knee
Adductors – longus, brevis & magnus	Pubis and ischium	Linea aspera and supra-condylar line	Adducts femur
Pectineus	Pubis	Close to lesser trochanter of femur	Adducts femur, flexes hip
Popliteus	Lateral condyle of femur	Tibia	Internally rotates and flexes the knee
Gastrocnemius	Medial and lateral condyles of femur	Through Achilles tendon to calcaneum	Plantarflexes the foot, flexes the knee
Soleus	Fibula and tibia	Calcaneum	Plantarflexes the foot
Peroneus longus	Tibia	Medial cuneiform and 1st metatarsal	Everts foot and plantarflexes ankle
Peroneus brevis	Tibia	5th metatarsal	Everts foot and plantarflexes the knee
Tibialis anterior	Shaft of tibia	Medial cuneiform and 1st metatarsal	Dorsiflexes and inverts the foot
Tibialis posterior	Tibia and fibula	Navicular and 2nd to 5th metatarsals	Inverts and plantarflexes the foot
Extensor digitorum longus	Tibia and fibula	Distal phalanges of toes	Extends toes, dorsiflexes the ankle and everts foot
Flexor digitorum longus	Posterior of tibia	Distal phalanges of toes	Flexes toes, plantarflexes the ankle and inverts foot

Myositis
Inflammation of a muscle.

Rupture
Burst or tear in the fascia or sheath surrounding muscles.

Spasm
A more than usual number of muscle fibres in sustained contraction, usually in response to pain. Fibres contract for much longer than is usually necessary.

Spasticity
This is caused when inhibitory nerves have been cut. Its effects are that spinal reflexes cause sustained contraction.

Sprain
A sudden twist or wrench of the joint's ligaments.

Strain
An over-stretching of a muscle, causing soreness and localised pain. May sometimes indicate a rupture (tear) in muscle fibres, tendon or fascia.

Stress
Stress is any factor which affects physical or mental well-being. Its effects are excessive muscle tension and subsequent muscle pain, especially in the back and neck.

You now know what the muscular system is, what it does and the types of diseases that affect it.

THE NERVOUS SYSTEM

What is it?
The nervous system is a communication and instruction network. It consists of two parts: the central nervous system (brain and spinal cord) and the peripheral nervous system (cranial nerves, spinal nerves, autonomic system including the parasympathetic and sympathetic nervous systems). The central nervous system controls the functions of the mind and behaviour as well as interpreting and reacting to the peripheral nervous system's messages; the peripheral nervous system controls our motor and sensory functions plus the action of the internal organs and sends information relating to them back to the brain.

What does it do?
The nervous system is one of the body's communication and instruction networks. The brain is the centre and it is connected to the rest of the body by nerve cells which carry information and instructions to and from it. When the brain is informed of danger, sensation or pain it can protect the body by sending out a warning. Thus, when a finger is placed in very hot water, the nerves send a message to the brain telling it that the water is too hot and may burn the skin and the brain sends a message telling the finger to move. We do not perceive this process because nerve impulses are involuntary and extremely fast.

Diseases of the nervous system
The nervous system can be stimulated by massage. Sufferers of severe nervous pain may find massage too painful and counterproductive over the affected areas but massage of related areas may be appropriate. Clients suffering from stress or mild nervous conditions may find it extremely helpful.

Bell's palsy
Facial paralysis, caused by injury to or infection of the facial nerve which subsequently becomes inflamed.

Motor neurone disease
A rare progressive disorder, in which the motor neurones in the body gradually deteriorate structurally and functionally.

Parkinson's disease
Progressive disease caused by damage to basal ganglia of the brain and resulting in loss of dopamine (neuro-transmitter). Causes tremor and rigidity in muscles, as well as difficulty and slowness with voluntary movement.

Stress
Such factors can be imagined, (e.g. worry about the future) or real, (e.g. financial problems). It is not the factor itself that is damaging but the response to it. Stress puts all the systems of the body on red alert, particularly the nervous system which tries to locate the danger, whether real or not, in order to tell the brain. This heightened activity causes symptoms such as churning stomach or 'butterflies', racing heart or palpitations, diarrhoea, loss of appetite, trembling, insomnia and sweating. Massage is extremely effective for treating stress because it stimulates the parasympathetic nervous system which slows down the action of some internal organs, particularly the heart.

Sciatica
Sciatica is often caused by the degeneration of an intervertebral disc which then causes pain in the lower back and the outside of the leg and foot. Massage is contraindicated over the affected area but soothing massage of the upper body may help relaxation and provide some pain relief.

Neuralgia
Stabbing pain along one or more nerves. Massage may be too painful over the affected area. Massage may also trigger neuralgia, which can be affected by light touch.

Neuritis
Inflammation of a nerve causing severe pain along it. Massage would be too painful over the affected area.

Myalgic encephalomyelitis (ME)
ME is also known as post-viral fatigue. Symptoms and suspected causes vary. It is characterised by extreme exhaustion which cannot be relieved by sleep or rest, general aches and pains, headaches and sometimes sore throat, fever, depression and swollen lymph nodes. Massage can sometimes provide a much needed dose of deep relaxation as well as an increased sense of well-being. It can also exhaust sufferers.

Multiple sclerosis
A disease which causes loss of the protective myelin sheath from nerve fibres in the central nervous system. Sufferers lose muscular coordination, sensation and have problems with speech and vision. Massage can help prevent spasm and stiffness in the muscles but the client should be referred before treatment.

You now know the basic structure and function of the skin, blood and lymph circulation, muscles and nerves and some of the diseases which affect them.

SUMMARY

- ***Massage is used over the whole surface of the body but is particularly beneficial for certain integral systems.***

3 Massage techniques

Learning objectives

The target knowledge of this chapter is:
- **massage techniques (classical/Swedish system)**
- **mediums used in massage.**

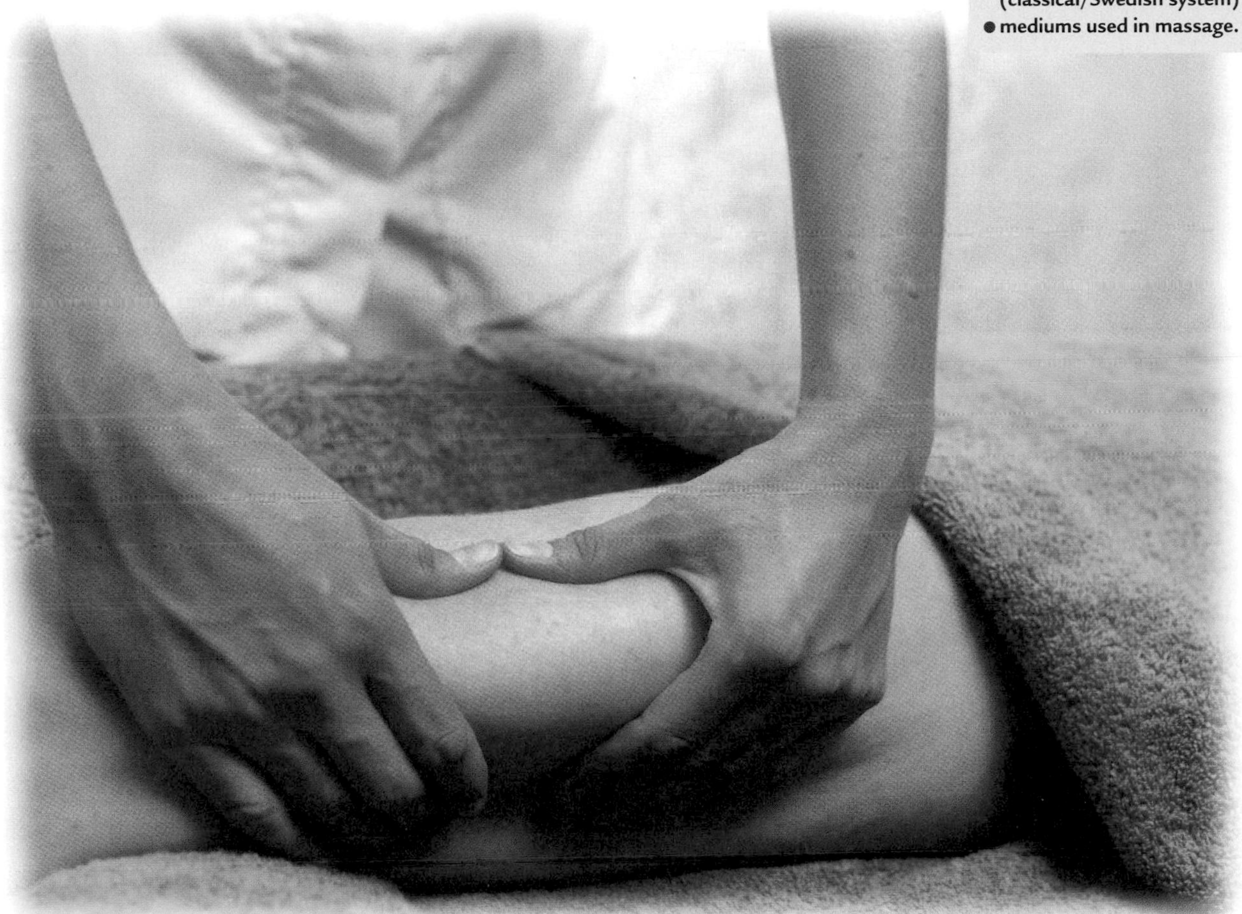

In Brief

Massage is the manipulation of muscles, leading to benefits for all the body systems. The techniques in this book, which are based on the Swedish system, use the application of pressure to either soothe or stimulate.

MASSAGE TECHNIQUES

What is massage?

Massage is a combination of various movements used to manipulate tissues for both local and overall effects and benefits. The movements range from gentle stroking to invigorating friction, depending on the desired effect. Massage is generally based on the Swedish system and several types of massage have developed which incorporate these techniques for different therapeutic effects.

What is Swedish massage?

The Swedish system of massage is named after the man who developed it, Per Henrik Ling. He was a physiologist and fencing master and developed a system of movements which he found helpful for improving his health and maintaining his physical condition. Classical massage is still based on the techniques he used, i.e. effleurage, petrissage and percussion. This chapter will look at these fundamental movements as well as variations of them.

EFFLEURAGE

What is effleurage?

The name effleurage derives from *effleurer*, a French word meaning 'to touch lightly'. It is generally a gentle, sweeping, relaxing stroke, with varying levels of pressure, used at the beginning and end of a massage. It can also be used with firm pressure over large areas once the muscles are relaxed. Unlike petrissage and percussion, effleurage does not aim to move or manipulate tissues or muscles, only to soothe and relax them and improve circulation.

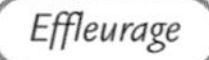
Effleurage

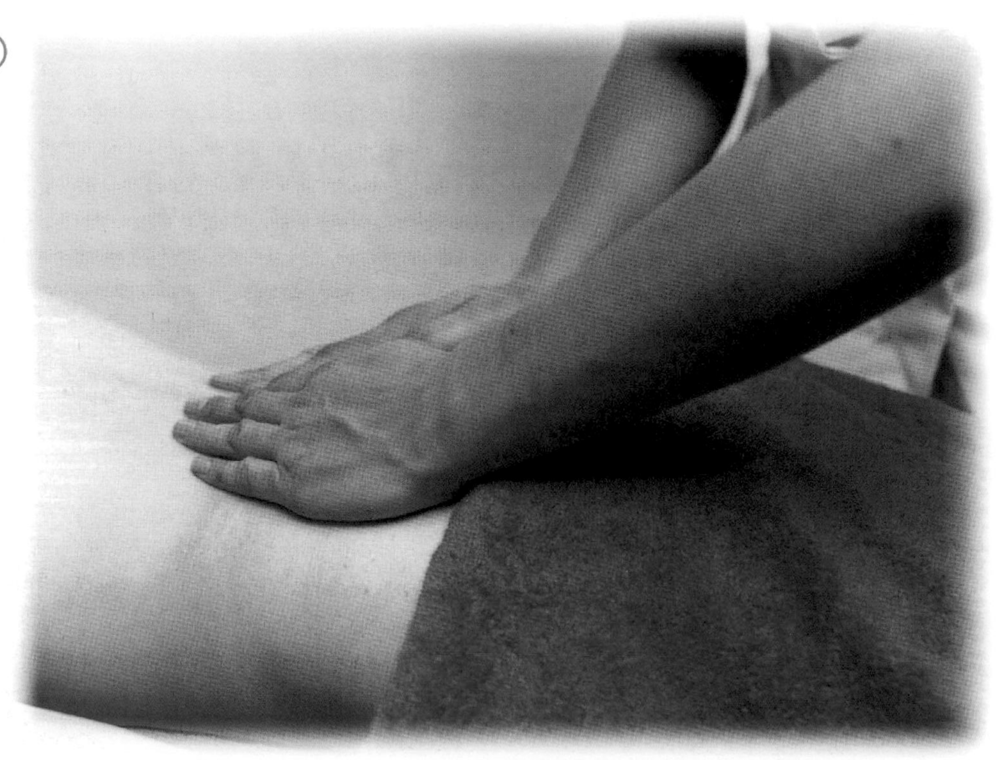

How to do it

With fingers and thumbs together, keep the hands relaxed and stroke the skin slowly and rhythmically with a confident pressure. When massaging the limbs, the emphasis of the pressure is towards the heart. The hands may be used one after the other or at the same time. The whole palm of the hand and the fingers should be used to prevent tickling the client. Hands must mould to the contours of the area being treated. Once a gentle rhythm has been established the therapist can increase the pressure gradually to prepare the body for the deeper work that follows.

If you remember only one thing...

Effleurage is a relaxing stroke that is used to prepare the body for deeper techniques.

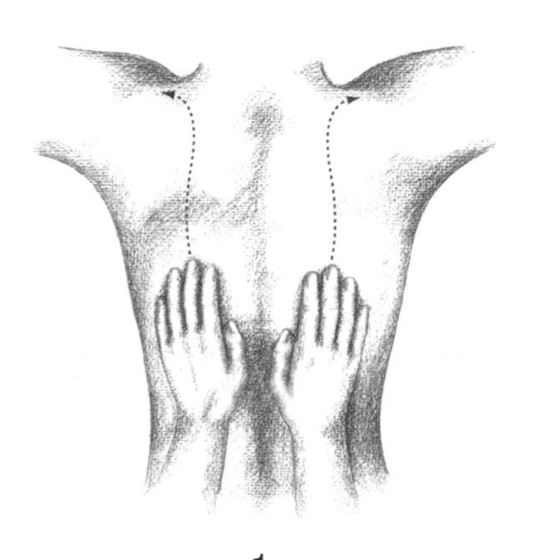
1

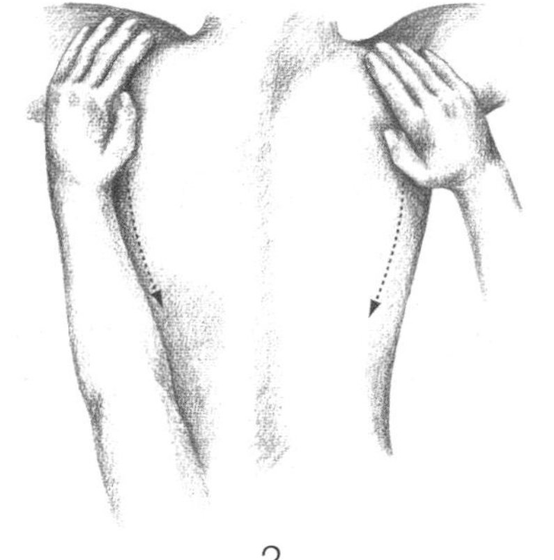
2

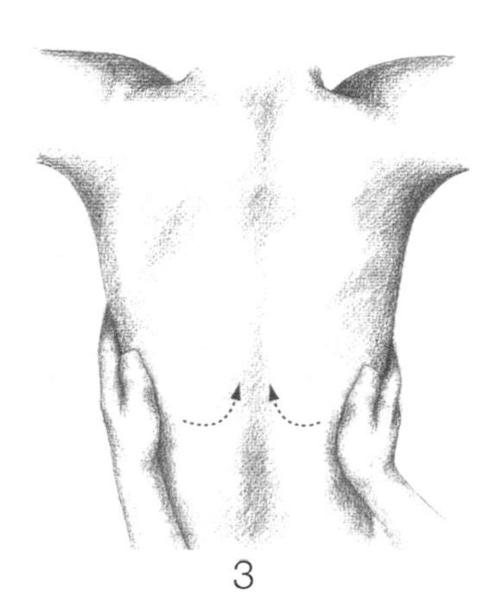
3

The three stages of effleurage (on the back)

When to use it

Effleurage is used at the start and finish of a massage session and at the start and finish of each body part, e.g. at the beginning and end of work on the back or legs. It is also used as a connection stroke between different parts of the massage. When carrying out a massage the therapist must not break contact with the client because when the hands are removed the client's body senses this, believes the massage is over and begins to rouse itself from its relaxed state.

Effleurage on the limbs with the pressure working towards the heart assists the return of blood to the heart and aids lymph drainage. Deep effleurage also pushes blood into superficial capillaries.

What does it do?

As the first contact between therapist and client, effleurage helps to prepare the body for massage, introducing the client to the therapist's touch, spreading the massage medium such as oil or cream (if used), warming the skin and relaxing the client. It is also used after more invigorating strokes to help the elimination of toxins from the areas that have been worked. It can also help desquamation, especially when used deeply, and thus help the skin to regenerate.

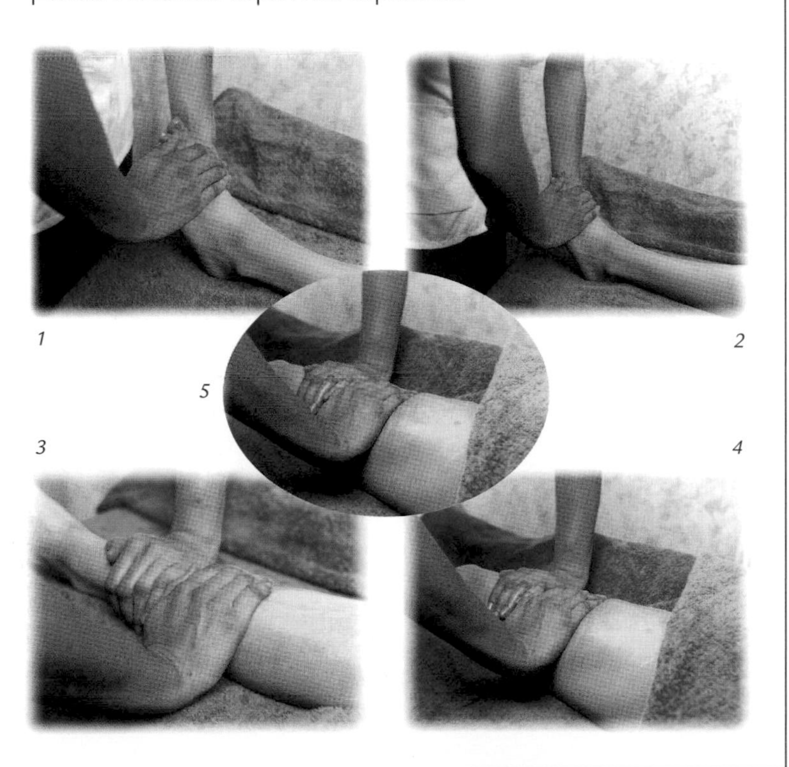
1 *2* *3* *4* *5*

PETRISSAGE

What is petrissage?

Petrissage, like effleurage, is a name deriving from French. *Pétrir* means to knead or rub with force and this stroke uses both kneading and rubbing movements to manipulate tissues and muscles. It uses the pressure of the hands or fingers to break down tension. There are various methods: in some cases only the fingers and/or thumbs are used to knead the tissues, in others the whole hand is used.

If you remember only one thing...

Petrissage (or kneading) is a firm application of pressure which compresses tissue against tissue, thus releasing muscle tightness and breaking down toxins and tension.

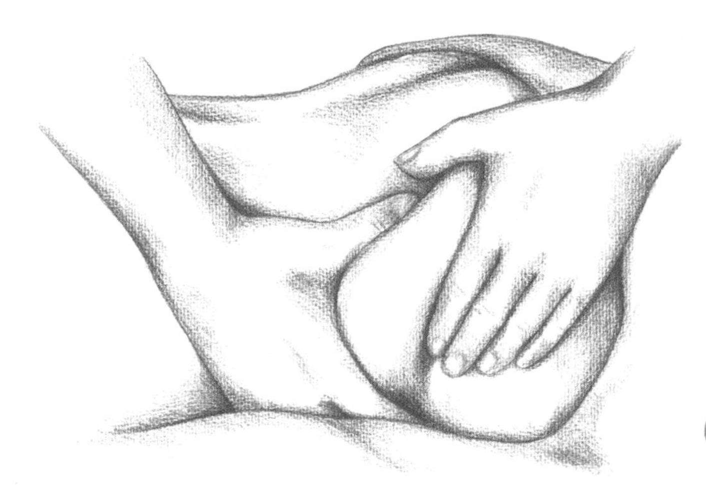

Kneading is a petrissage stroke

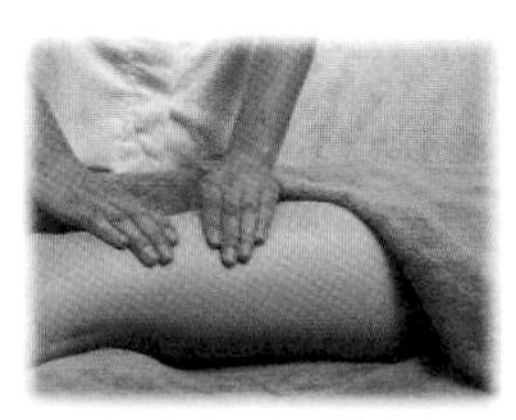

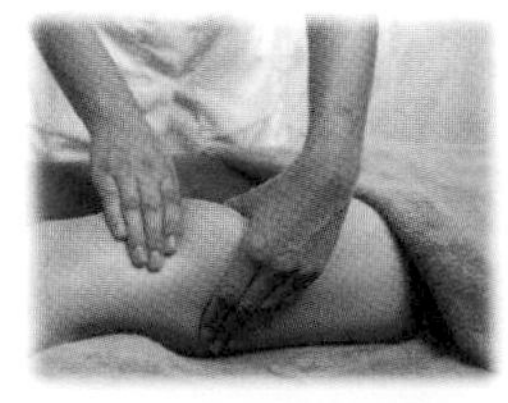

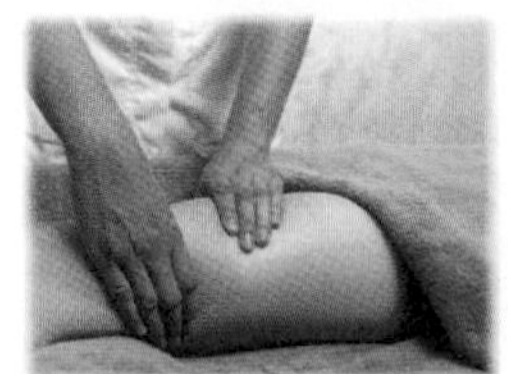

How to do it

Carefully and slowly grasp the flesh of the part of the body being worked with both hands or fingers then use one hand to lift it, as if pulling it away from the bone. Keep the tissues firmly compressed whilst lifting, then release and repeat with the other hand. Continue to lift, compress and release with alternate hands, as if kneading dough and build up into a rhythm. For particularly stiff/tight areas, build a twist into the movement so that the flesh is being 'wrung' like a damp cloth. The pressure should be smooth and not jerky and care should be taken to avoid pinching the skin. Begin gently and build up to firmer pressure, always using the same rate and rhythm and getting feedback from the client. It is important to use body weight and movement to assist in making the technique effective and less tiring for the therapist. Lean into the muscle as you grasp it and lean back as you lift.

When to use it

Petrissage usually follows effleurage at the start of a massage. It should be used to break down tightness and tension in large muscles. It should not be used on bony or delicate areas.

What does it do?

Petrissage stretches the muscles, improving their suppleness and elasticity, and helps break down tension and stiffness in tissues and large muscles. Such stiffness is often caused by the build-up of toxins such as lactic acid. Petrissage helps to release and break down these toxins, enabling the muscles to work more efficiently. It also stimulates the circulation and is very useful in sports massage. Despite the firmness of the stroke it is more relaxing than invigorating because it releases any tight muscles and the toxins within.

FRICTION

The name friction, like many others used in massage, comes from a Latin word, *fricare*, which means to rub or rub down. Friction techniques are all variations of rubbing and they work by compressing tissue against bone. It is often used for close work on a small area or on specific areas of tightness.

How to do it

Place thumbs or fingers, particularly the balls/pads of the thumb, on the section of the body to be worked. Apply firm pressure from your body and circle the tissue immediately below the thumbs slowly and deeply. Try to imagine the tissues below the surface of the skin and how the rubbing movement pushes them against other muscles and against the bones creating friction. The thumbs can be rubbed up and down or held in a static position. Fingertips can also be used if the therapist finds them more effective. Once the small area has been thoroughly worked move to another section. The therapist should not be moving rapidly across an expanse of flesh but deliberately and slowly focusing on a small section at a time, moving along the length of a muscle. Depending on the type of skin/ individual's requirements the therapist will need to adjust the length of time spent on each small area in order to prevent rubbing for too long and causing soreness. The effect should be one of heat and tension.

Cross-fibre friction is a variation of this technique in which the therapist works across the muscle at right angles to the fibres instead of along the length of the muscle. This helps to stretch the muscle fibres and release tension. It is used extensively by physiotherapists and sports massage therapists in the treatment of injuries.

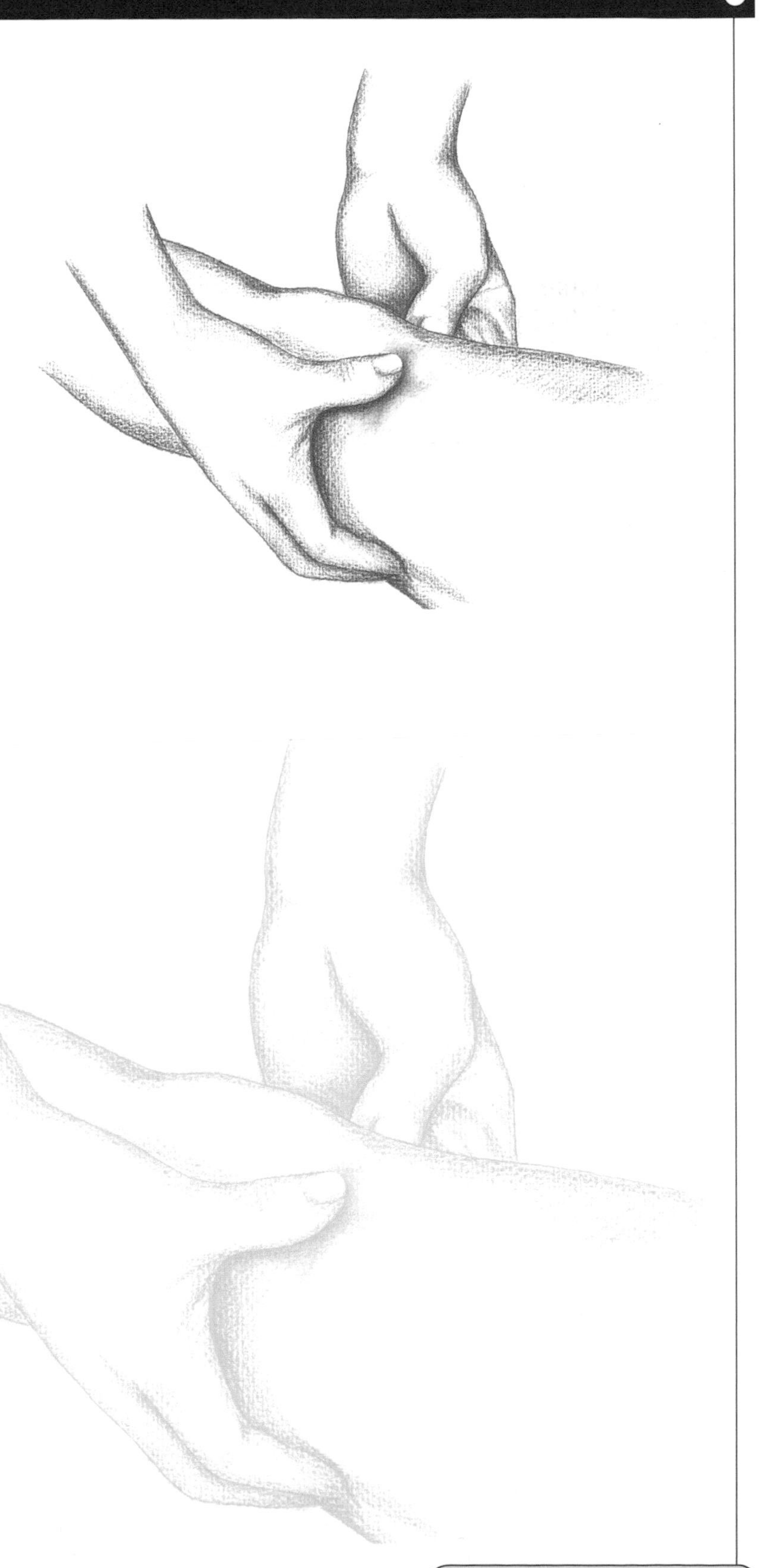

When to use it

Friction is a method used for focusing on a particular problem area. It is especially useful for releasing tension in muscles and for loosening tightness around joints. It is not recommended for use all over the body because it is time-consuming and tiring for the therapist. It is also used on small muscles where petrissage is not appropriate. On tight muscles friction can be very painful, so caution is vital in the care of the client.

What does it do?

Friction movements heat up the local area, improve circulation, promote lymph drainage, stimulate the nerves and loosen tightness in the muscles. Working very closely with the muscles helps to break down any local 'knottiness' or lumpiness. Cross-fibre friction helps stretch the muscle fibres and release any tension held in the muscle; it also allows the therapist, particularly in sports massage, to work close to a damaged or inflamed area without touching it, because working on one section of muscle helps stretch the rest of the muscle.

If you remember only one thing...

Frictions are firm rubbing and heat-producing techniques which compress tissue against bone. They are used for close work on areas of tension or by physiotherapists or sports massage therapists in treating injury.

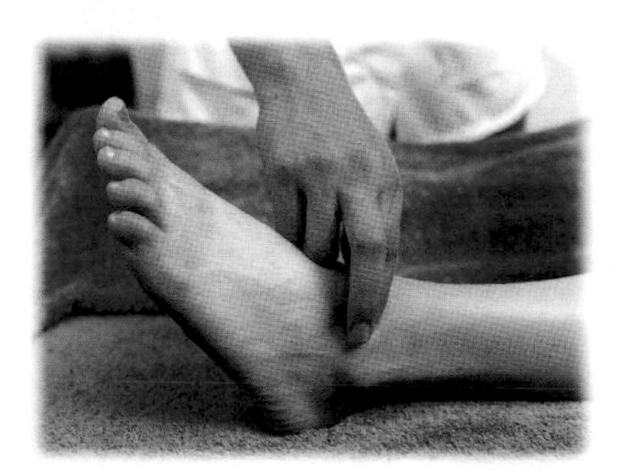

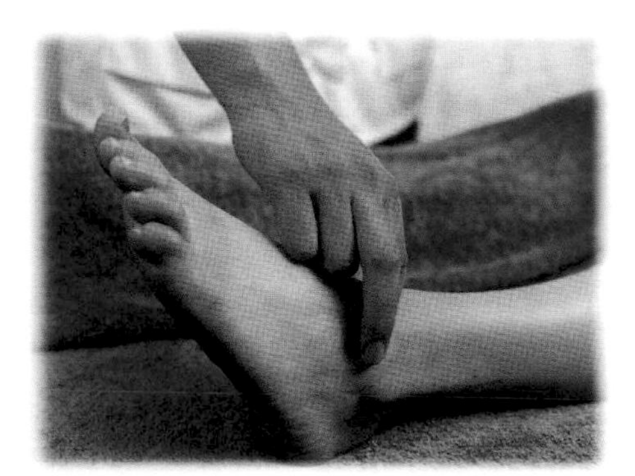

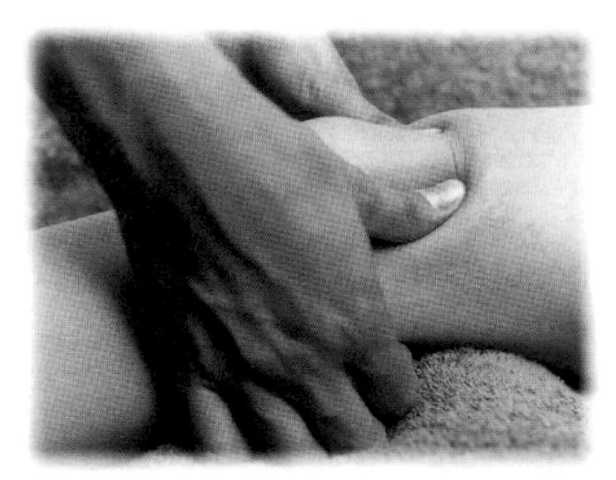

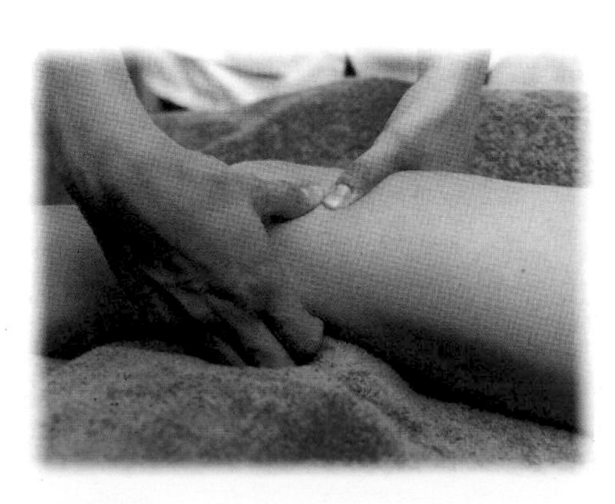

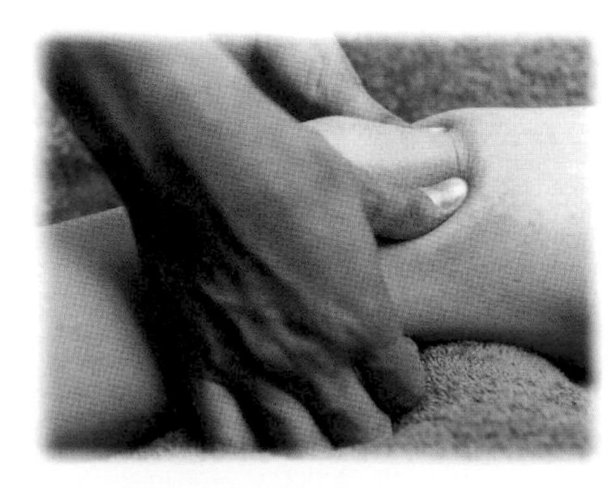

PERCUSSION

What is percussion?

Percussion derives from the Latin word *percutere* meaning to hit. Percussion techniques are brisk, invigorating and stimulating strokes, which use the hands to strike the body rapidly and suddenly. The classic 'chopping' motion associated with Swedish massage is a percussion technique called hacking. The others are pounding, beating, cupping and tapotement.

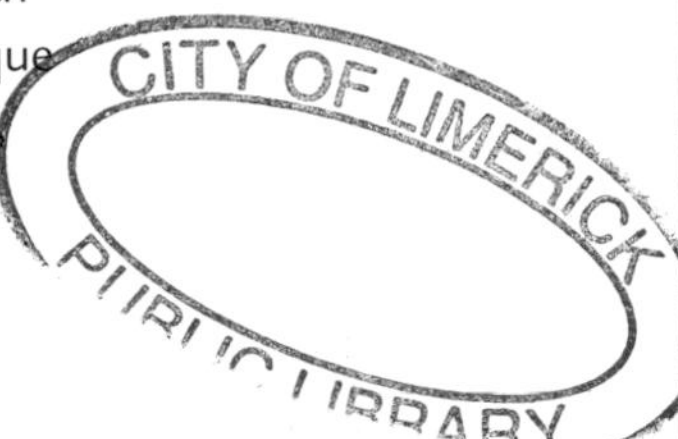

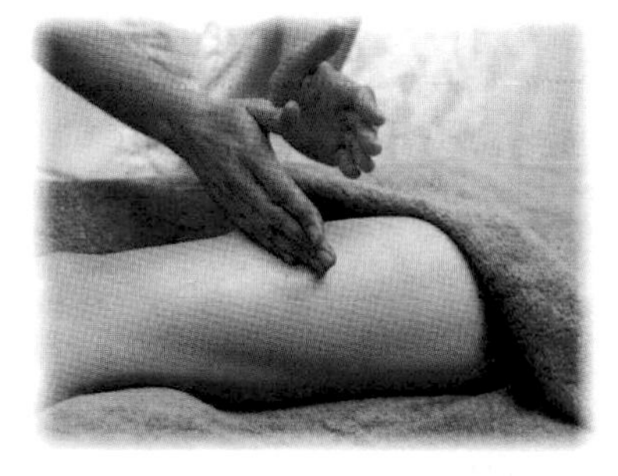

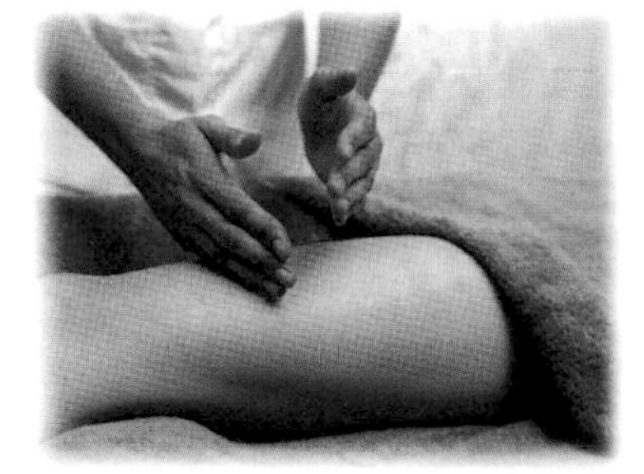

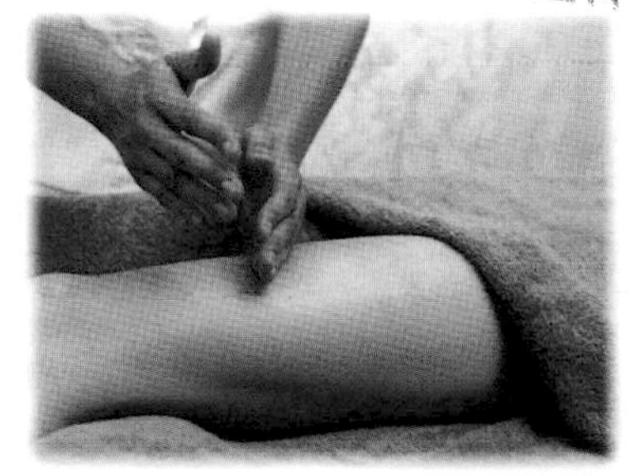

A classic massage technique called hacking

How to do it

Hacking: hold both hands over the body with palms facing each other and the edge of the little finger closest to the client. The fingers should be open and the elbows out, away from the body. Strike the body with alternate hands, with the movement originating from the wrist. As soon as one hand touches the skin let it spring back as the other drops to hack. Begin slowly with a light pressure and build up to a vigorous rhythm with firm pressure. Keep the hands and wrists relaxed to prevent causing pain and keep the rhythm bouncy and light.

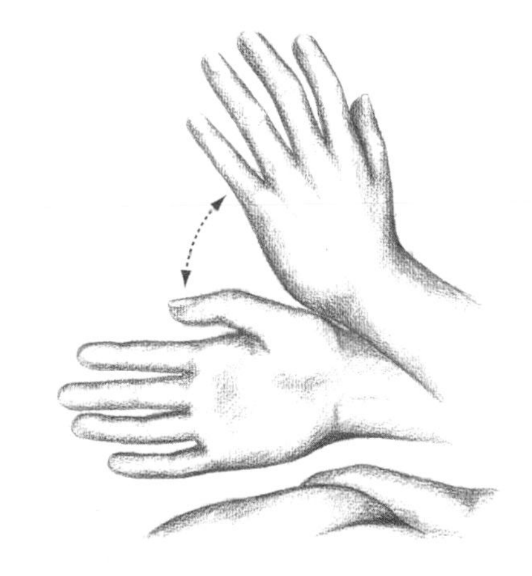

Pounding: make hands into fists, with the little finger side facing down towards the client's skin. Lower one fist then the other alternately, lifting one fist as the other lowers. Begin slowly with a light pressure and build up to a vigorous rhythm with firm pressure. Keep both hands and wrists relaxed and keep the movement brisk and springy so that the fists bounce away from the body as soon as they touch it and do not thump or cause pain. Pounding should only be used on fleshy areas.

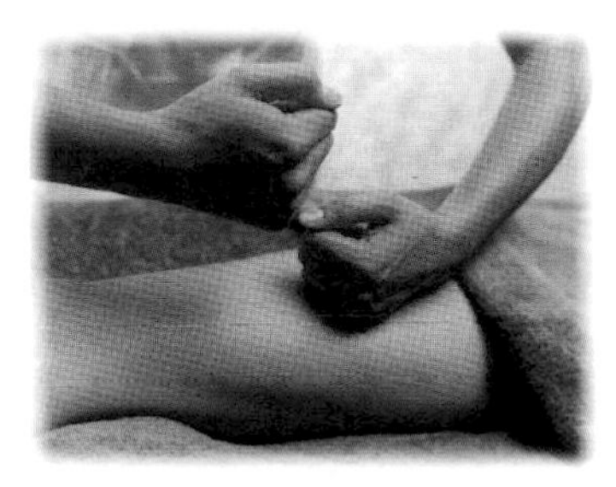

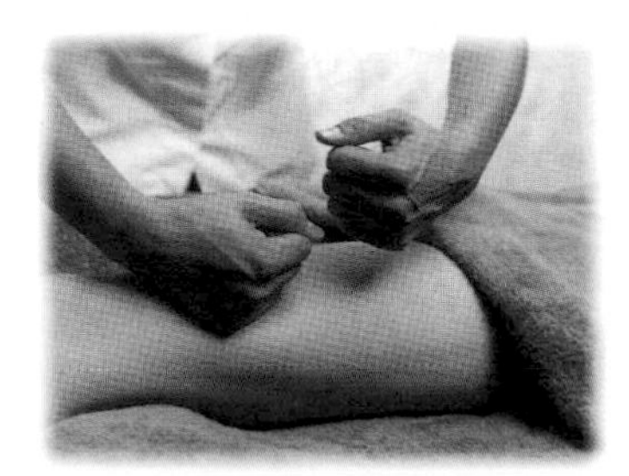

Did you know?

Percutere **(the origin of the word percussion) can be broken down into** ***per*** **meaning through and** ***quatere*** **means to shake. Percussion thus means a shaking through the body.**

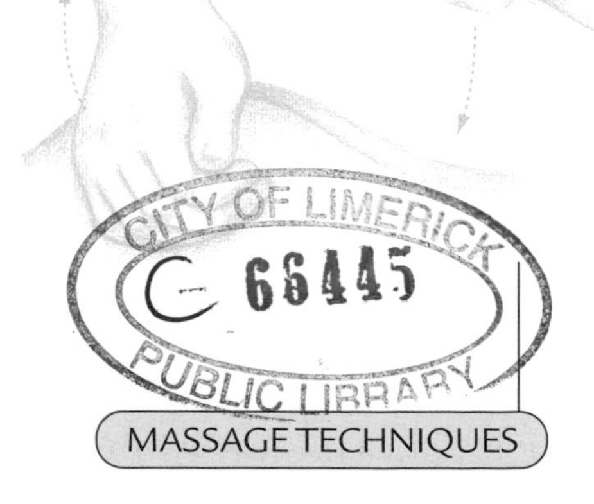

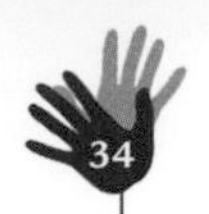

Beating: Similar to pounding except the knuckles of the fist hit the tissue rather than the side of the fist.

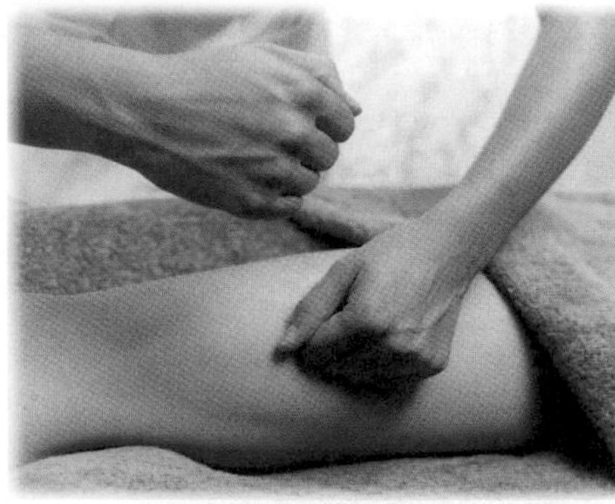

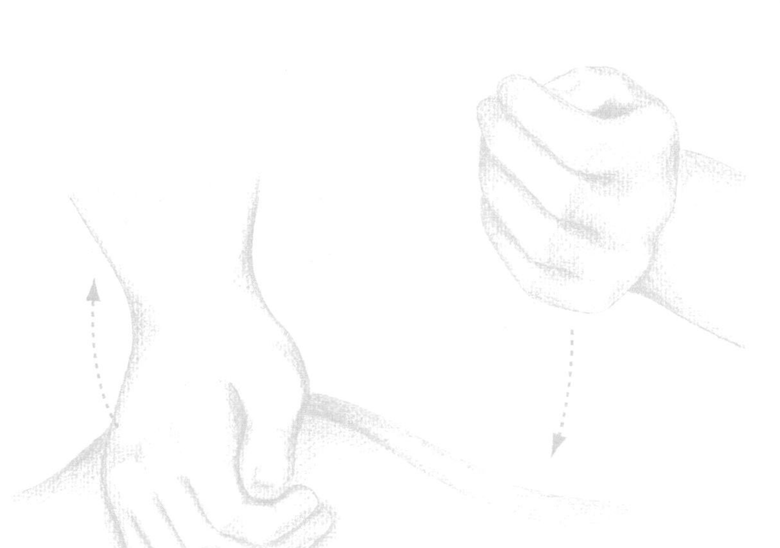

Pounding

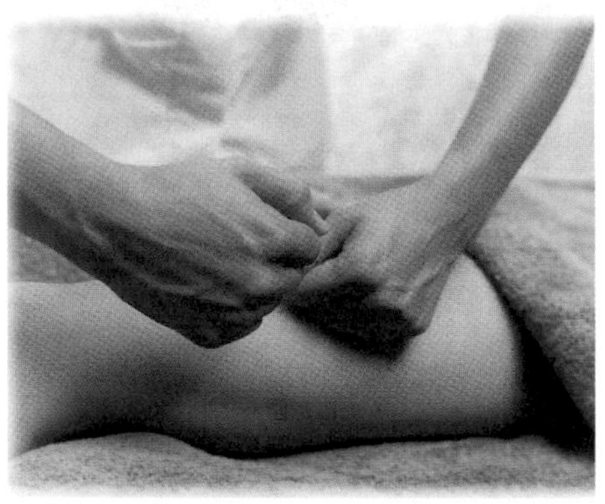

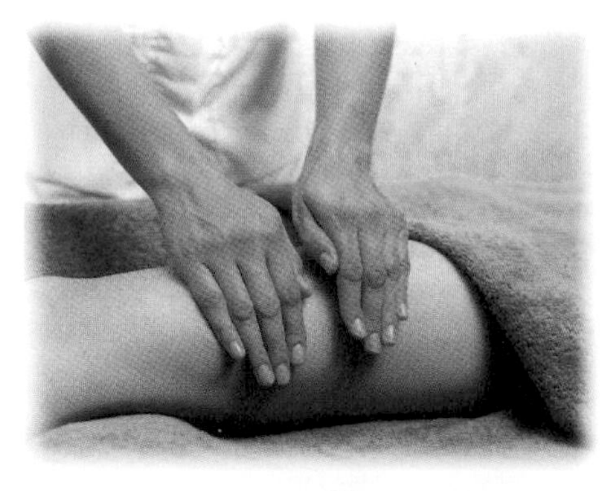

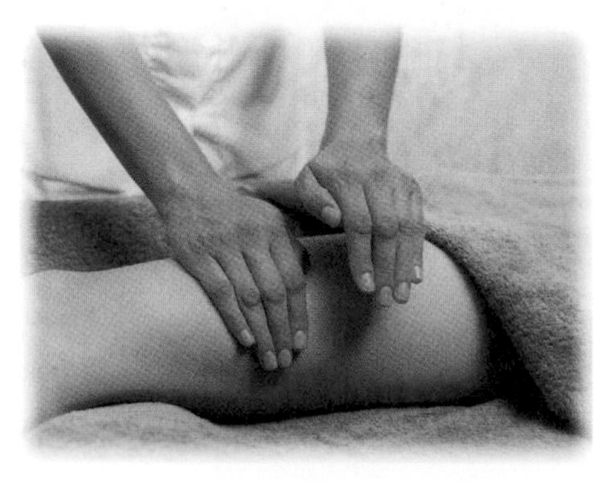

Cupping: hold hands out with palm facing up then form 'cup' shapes with the hands. Invert the 'cups' so that the 'inside' is closest to the client's skin. Then, following the same rhythm as hacking, lower one 'cup' then the next alternately. Begin slowly with light pressure and build up to a vigorous rhythm with firm pressure. Keep both hands and wrists relaxed and keep the movement brisk and springy. If done properly, the movement will create a 'popping' sound as air is pushed away from the surface of the skin by the pressure of the cupped hands, thus creating a vacuum. Be careful not to slap. It is the coming off the body with suction that stimulates the systems of the body, particularly the cardiovascular system. A redness, or erythema, may develop.

Tapotement: this is a very gentle form of percussion, using just the fingertips, which is carried out on delicate or sensitive areas, such as the face. The name derives from *tapoter*, a French word meaning to tap, and tapping is the basis of the technique. Keep the fingers loose and relaxed and tap the area very lightly and gently. Start slowly and build up to a gentle, repetitive and firm rhythm. As with other percussion movements the hands should be relaxed in order to keep the stroke bouncy. This is a soothing movement and should not be heavy or jerky.

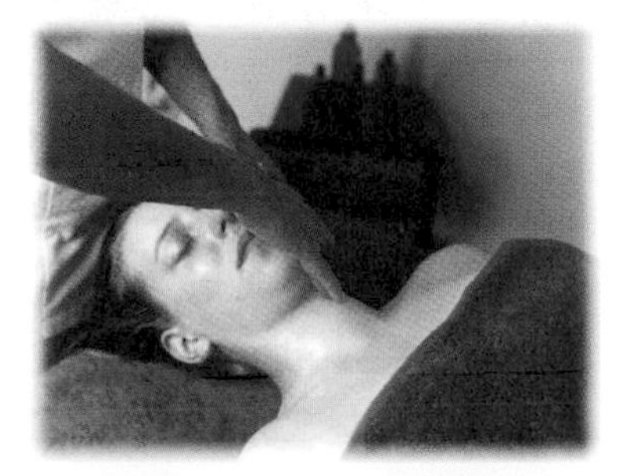
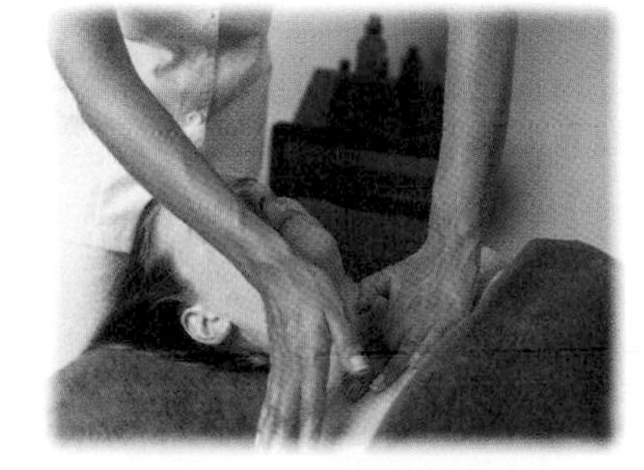
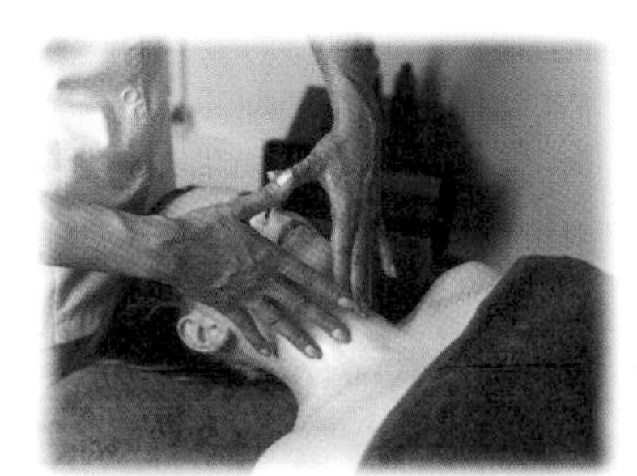
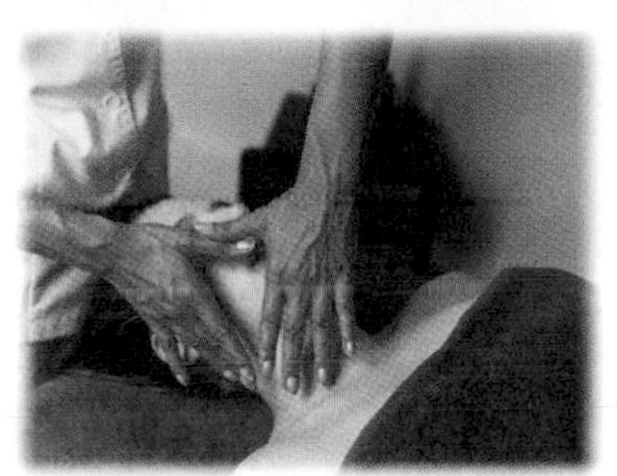
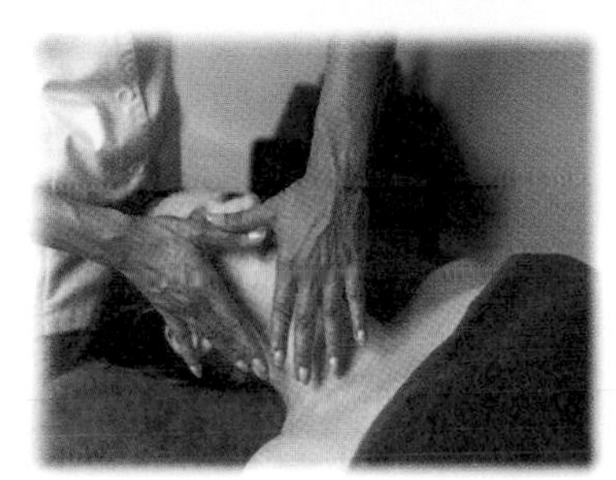
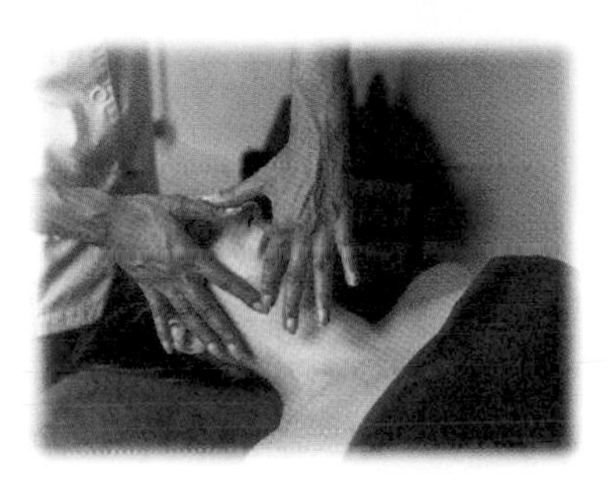

When to use it

Percussion should be used as an invigorating, wake-up stroke. If the aim of the whole massage is to stimulate the system rather than soothe it, percussion should form the major part of the treatment. If the aim of the massage is to soothe or relax, percussion can be used towards the end of the treatment, before the final effleurage strokes, to 'wake up' the client's systems. It should not be used on bony or delicate areas.

What does it do?

Percussion is the most invigorating of massage techniques. It improves local and overall circulation, warms the skin and muscles, improves muscle tone both because of the physical effect of the treatment and because of the improved circulation, helps break up fat deposits in fleshy areas and invigorates the nerves.

If you remember only one thing...

Percussion is a striking, wake-up stroke. It has a stimulating action on the tissues.

You now know the classic Swedish massage techniques, how to use them and why. The next section explains other massage techniques.

OTHER TECHNIQUES

If you remember only one thing...

Vibration is a pain reliever which clears nerve pathways and helps loosen tightness in the muscles.

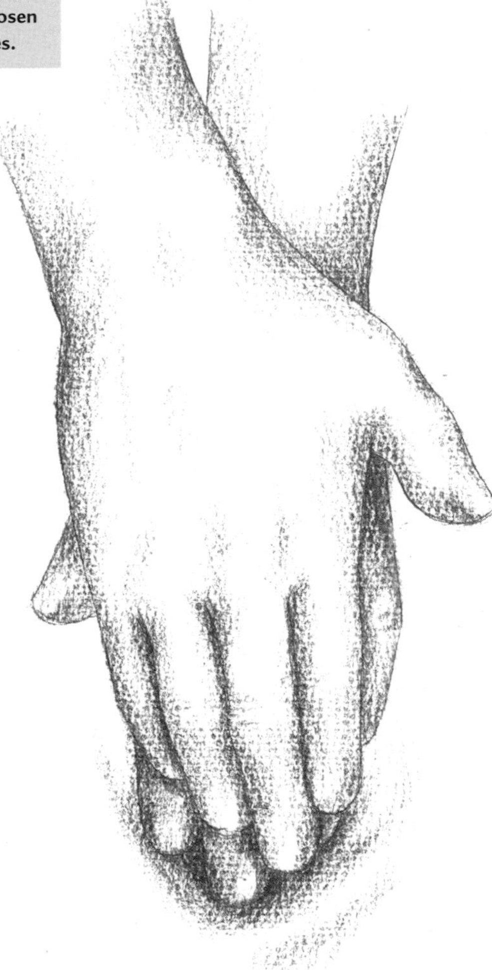

What is vibration?

Vibration can be either manual or mechanical. It aims to make the muscle tremble and shake in order to loosen tightness and release tension. Mechanical vibration equipment can be used to produce the same effects.

How to do it

Vibration can be carried out using either one or both hands and either whole palms or just the fingertips. Place the palms of the hands/fingertips on the muscle and, retaining firm, deep contact with the muscle throughout the movement, briskly move the hands/fingertips up and down or from side to side.

When to use it

When muscles are extremely tight and not responding well to petrissage or frictions.

What does it do?

Vibration helps release pain and tension. It can be a very soothing technique or a very stimulating one, depending on the desired result. It can literally surprise the muscle into releasing its tension.

Passive joint movements

Passive movements require the client to relax and let the therapist gently take a joint (e.g. knee, elbow, shoulder) through its natural range of movement. These movements may help to improve mobility and release tension.

REMEMBER

- Massage movements should always be used with upward pressure towards the heart. This helps venous return and lymphatic drainage.
- During a massage session the therapist should always aim to keep at least one hand in contact with the client, to prevent interrupting the mood of relaxation, and to reassure the client.
- Percussion and petrissage should not be used on bony or delicate areas.
- The therapist should start with light strokes and gentle pressure and build up to deeper strokes and firmer pressure, whilst maintaining a slow rate and rhythm throughout.

GENERAL SUMMARY

Massage techniques and effects

The following is a general summary of the styles of movement or pressure used in massage and their effects on the body. It is intended as a guideline, not an absolute. With some treatments and some clients different effects may result and the styles may be used differently.

- **Superficial movement:** soothing, relaxing, preparatory, concluding.
- **Gentle movement:** soothing, relaxing, preparatory and concluding over delicate, sensitive, painful areas.
- **Deep movement:** relaxing, tension-release, pain reliever over muscular areas.
- **Brisk movement:** stimulating, pain reliever over muscular areas.
- **Light pressure:** stimulating over sensitive, painful areas.
- **Firm pressure:** relaxing, tension-release, pain reliever over muscular areas.
- **Slow movement:** soothing, relaxing, preparatory, concluding over delicate, sensitive, painful areas.
- **Fast movement:** stimulating, pain reliever over muscular areas.

How do I use the techniques in a routine?

The therapist's routine

Per Ling used the following routine: effleurage, petrissage, effleurage, percussion, effleurage. However, all massage therapists will develop their own routines according to the requirements of their clients. The therapist is the source of the massage and thus can control its effects and results. It is the therapist's responsibility to find out about the client's requirements and expectations and plan a routine that will meet them. For example, a client who wants a thorough, invigorating massage will require a routine built around stimulating techniques such as percussion with less focus on relaxing, gentle strokes like effleurage. A client who wants a relaxing massage will require a routine that focuses on effleurage and petrissage with less emphasis on percussion, if it is used at all. Mechanical methods are generally not used in relaxation because they are not as effective as the hands, either for palpating the muscles or for relaxing the client through touch. The time spent on each type of movement and the pressure used will also be determined by the individual's needs and the desired results.

The client's input

Each individual will experience massage techniques differently so that one may find a percussion movement very invigorating whereas another finds it painful. Again the therapist must work with the client to achieve the best results. The aim is to invigorate and/or soothe and at no time should the client's comments, especially with respect to pain, be ignored. The therapist must learn to adapt to each client's pain threshold. Ignoring it will in the short-term prevent the massage from being relaxing and in the long-term may cause damage.

Why are continuous movements necessary?

One hand or both should always be kept on the body during treatment since as soon as the hands are removed the body will register this as the end of the massage and begin to 'change gear', getting ready to dress and leave.

You now know the different techniques used in massage, how and when to perform them and what they do. You also know the importance of the therapist's input and that of the client. The next section explains what a massage medium is and why it is used.

MASSAGE MEDIUMS

What is a massage medium?
A massage medium is a lubricant which helps the therapist's hands to move freely and smoothly over the client's skin. The three most common mediums used are oil, cream and talc.

Massage oils
Oil is the most useful massage medium because it is smooth and light. Massage oils should be of vegetable or plant origin and not too thick or heavy because the heat and pressure of massage movements can make them sticky. Lighter oils, such as grapeseed, are more useful for larger areas because they are smoother. Thicker oils, such as avocado are more useful for smaller areas. Blends of oils can be used either for a blend of properties or to make a more expensive oil go further, e.g. a dense, expensive oil such as evening primrose oil, which is very good for use on dry skin, could be blended with a lighter, less expensive oil such as grapeseed. Mineral oils, such as baby oil, should not be used as they dry the skin.

See Chapter 7 for more information on using oils in aromatherapy massage.

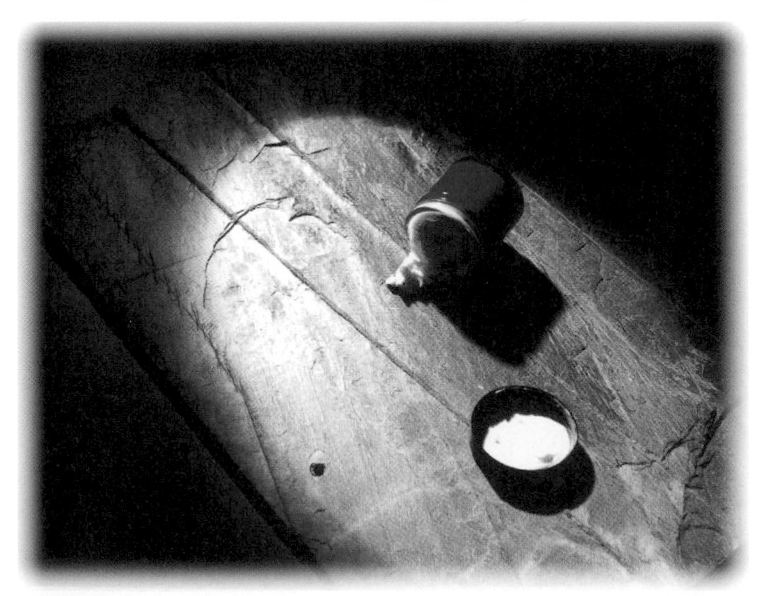

Massage creams
Creams are good for small or delicate areas such as the face or on very dry skin. They tend to be heavier and greasier than oils. As they are absorbed faster than massage oils, they may require more frequent application.

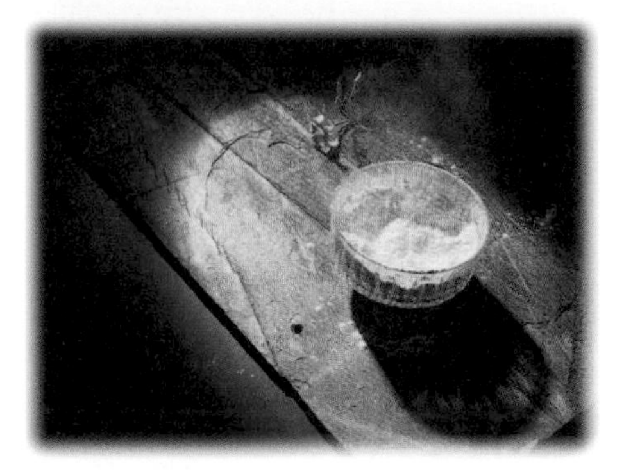

Talcum powder
Talcum powder is useful for oily skin, very hairy clients or on clients who dislike the residues of oils and creams. Swedish massage was traditionally performed using talc because talc prevents the hands from sliding over the surface of the body and allows deeper pressure.

How much medium should I use?
The amount of medium used will depend on the client. In general a full body massage will require about 20-25 ml of oil. Massage of larger clients and those with dry skin will require more medium.

How do I apply it?
All massage mediums should first be dispensed into the therapist's hands, rather than straight on to the client's body. This is because the oil, cream or powder will be cold and uncomfortable on the skin if it is not warmed up and evenly distributed. The therapist should dispense a small amount into the palm of one hand and then rub the hands together to warm the medium and distribute it smoothly across palms and fingertips. The

therapist should then apply the medium using effleurage strokes.

Sensitive skin and allergies

Before using any oil, cream or talcum powder, the therapist may wish to carry out a patch test, especially if the client has sensitive skin or allergies. Wash the crook of the elbow with water or water and a mild soap, dry it then rub a small amount of the medium onto the skin. Leave for 24 hours and check for any reactions.

You now know the different techniques and mediums used in massage.

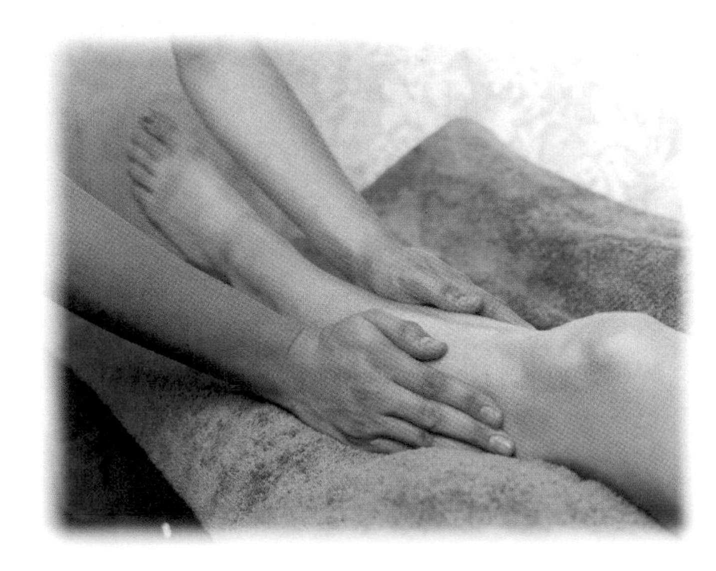

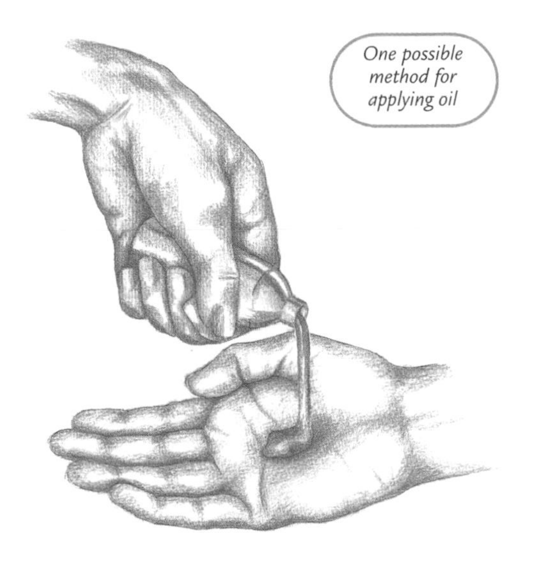

One possible method for applying oil

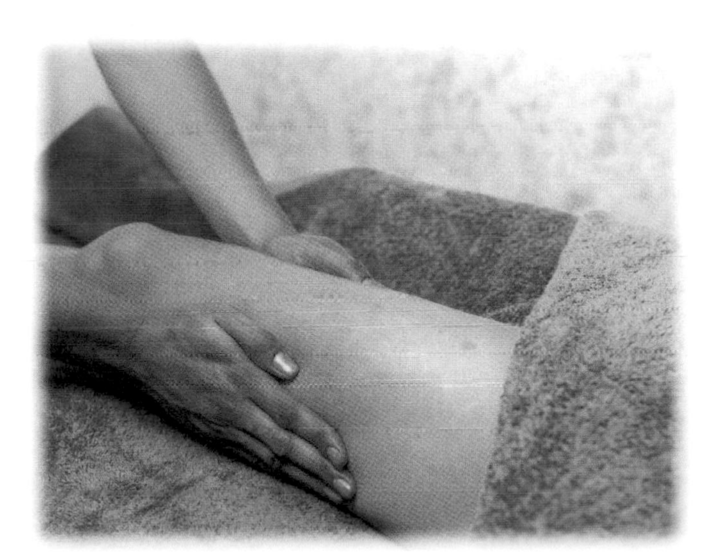

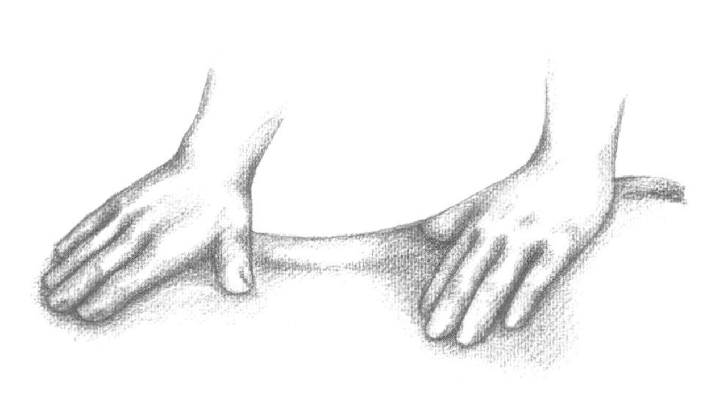

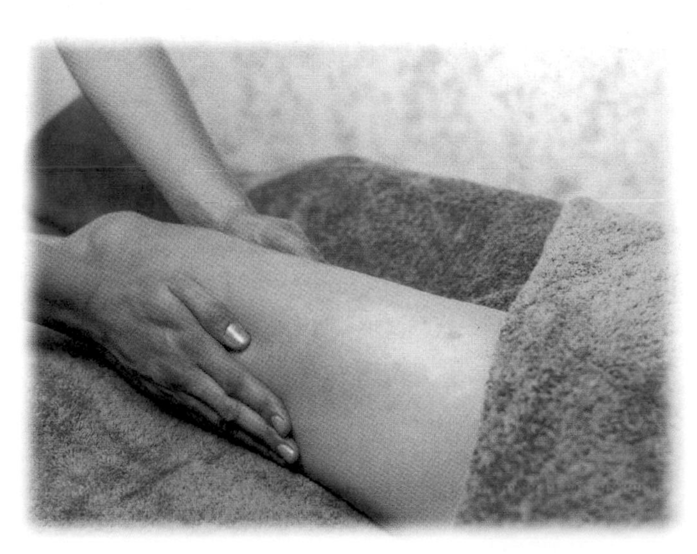

4 Effects and benefits of massage

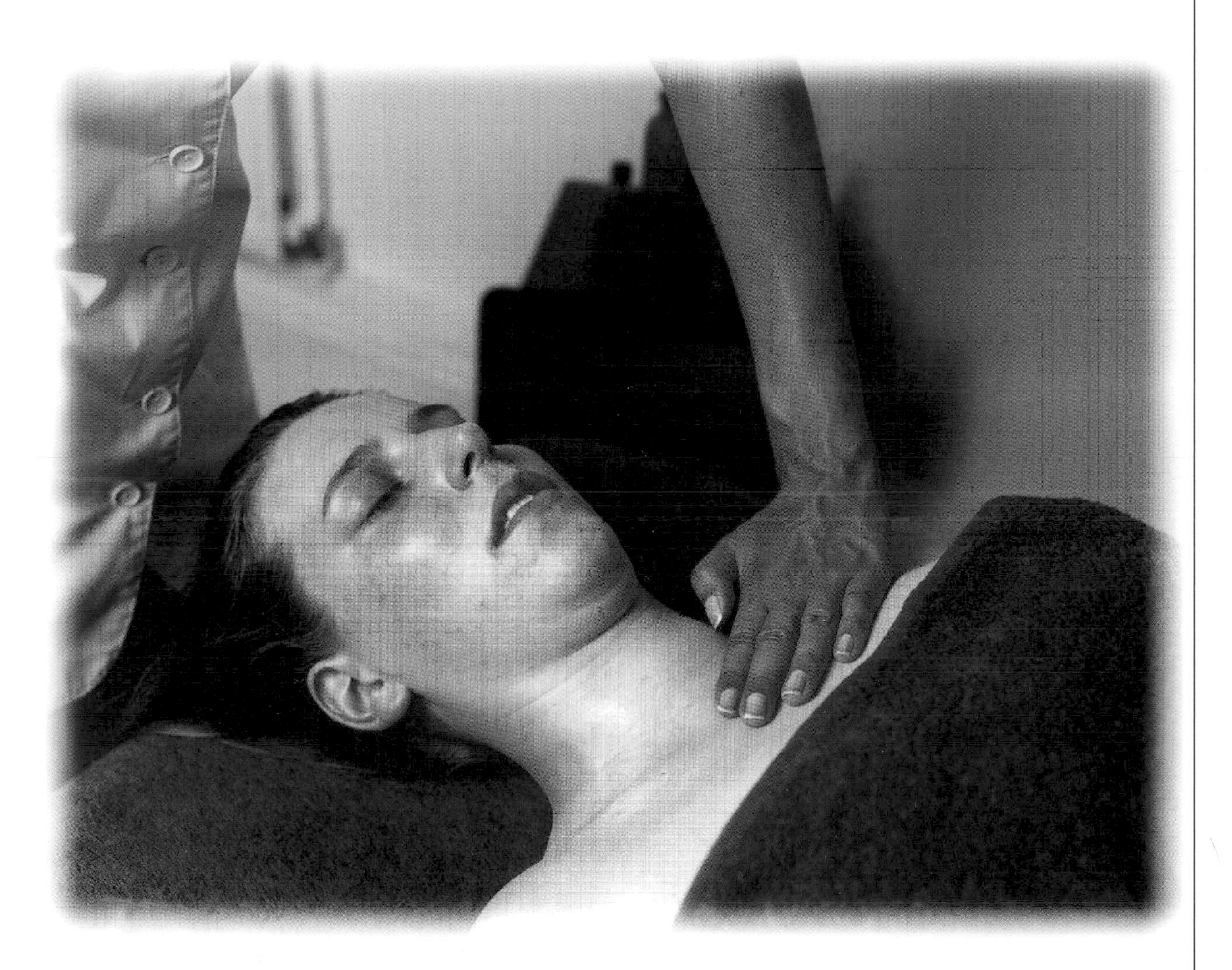

In Brief

Massage has an immediate local and physiological effect on the part of the body being worked and it also affects the whole body through stimulation and relaxation of the nerves. It has physiological and psychological benefits and can affect all of the body systems in a positive way.

Learning objectives

The target knowledge of this chapter is:

- physiological effects and benefits of massage
- psychological effects and benefits of massage
- effects of massage on different body systems.

THE EFFECTS AND BENEFITS OF MASSAGE

What are the effects of massage?

The effects of massage are twofold: physiological (relating to the physical structure of the body) and psychological (relating to the mind). When the body is massaged, the mechanics (i.e. the physical action of manipulating tissue) affect the local area of the massage, whereas the nervous stimulation (i.e. the response of the nerves to touch and movement), affects the whole body. Evidently the positive benefits of massage for the physical body will affect the psychological body and vice-versa. However, for the purposes of study they have been divided into physiological and psychological.

Physiological

In the short term massage will:

- improve skin tone and colour by removing dead cells (desquamating) and improving circulation
- encourage better circulation therefore more efficient delivery of nutrients and oxygen to cells and more efficient waste removal
- encourage deeper and therefore more efficient and relaxed breathing
- encourage better lymph drainage and reduce swelling
- relieve muscle fatigue, soreness and stiffness
- relieve tired, stiff joints
- promote general relaxation
- sedate or stimulate the nervous system (depending on type of massage performed)
- encourage sleep
- speed up digestion and waste removal.

In the long term massage will:

- improve skin elasticity
- improve circulation
- boost immunity
- improve muscle suppleness
- improve neural communication and relax the nervous system (preventing, for example, muscle spasms caused by anxiety)
- enable deeper, more effective respiration
- relieve insomnia
- balance the digestive system
- lower high blood pressure.

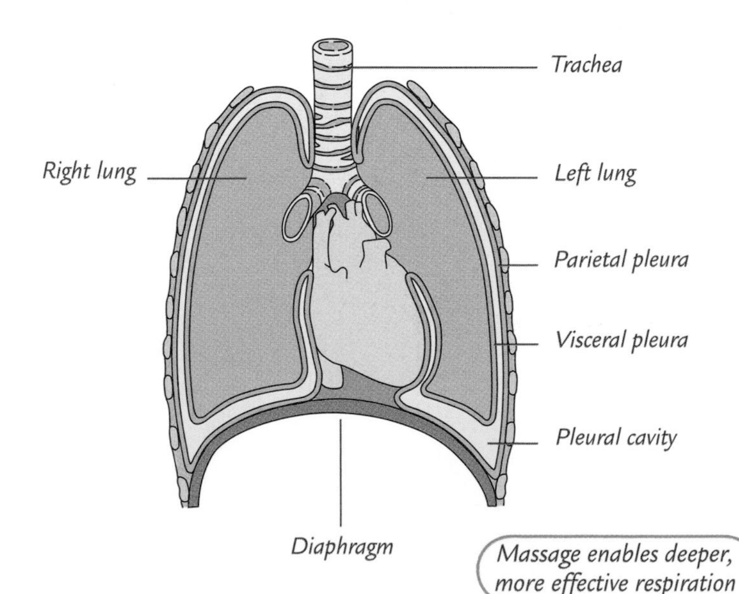

Massage enables deeper, more effective respiration

Psychological

In the short term massage will:

- relax the body, thereby reducing tension and the effects of stress
- relax the mind, thereby reducing anxiety and its effects
- soothe and comfort the client
- give a 'lift' to the emotions and increase positive feelings
- increase energy by invigorating all body systems and reducing fatigue.

In the long term massage will:

- enable sustained relaxation of body and mind
- improve body image, awareness and general self-esteem
- increase energy levels less energy is spent in holding the body in a state of tension and strain (both physical and mental).

THE SYSTEMS OF THE BODY

The first part of this section explains the effects of massage on the systems that are directly affected. The second part explains the effects on systems that benefit more indirectly.

The cell

Although when a massage is carried out it is not necessary to think of every cell and the effects on it, it helps to recognise that what happens on a global level in a massage also happens at a cellular level. Since massage improves the workings of, and invigorates, body systems, it has the same effect at a cellular level. The delivery of nutrients, oxygen and water, and the removal of carbon dioxide, toxins and waste is faster and more efficient, digestion and respiration are improved and each cell can therefore work at its optimum level.

A single cell (generalised)

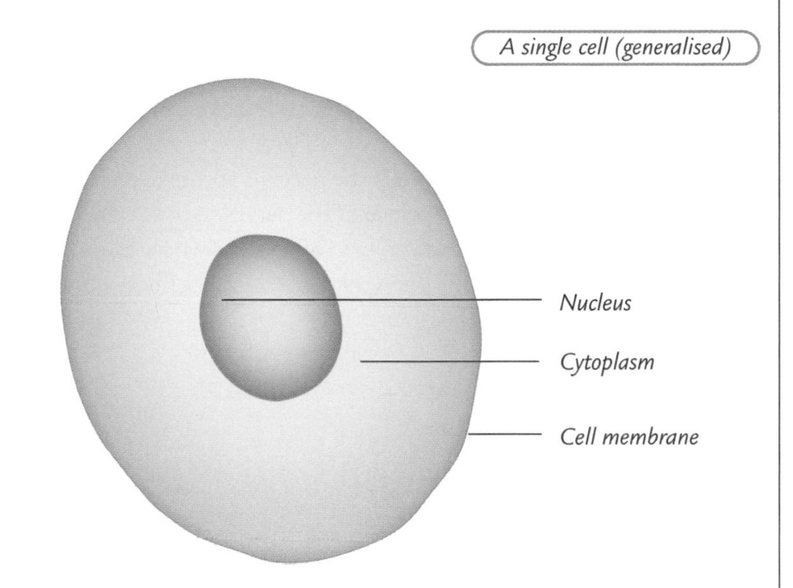

The skin

The skin is the most obvious part of the body to benefit from massage. The therapist is in constant contact with it throughout the duration of the massage and this not only invigorates the skin but also soothes and relaxes the client.

The effects of massage include:

- **improved skin colour:** poor skin colour is often associated with poor circulation; massage boosts the circulation and thus invigorates skin colour;
- **improved skin tone and texture:** the constant stroking and rubbing of the skin helps speed up desquamation (the removal of dead skin cells) and this encourages the regeneration of the skin cells and better tone;
- **improved elasticity:** massage encourages the production of sebum, the skin's natural oil, which helps keep the skin lubricated and prevents dryness.

Cross-section of skin

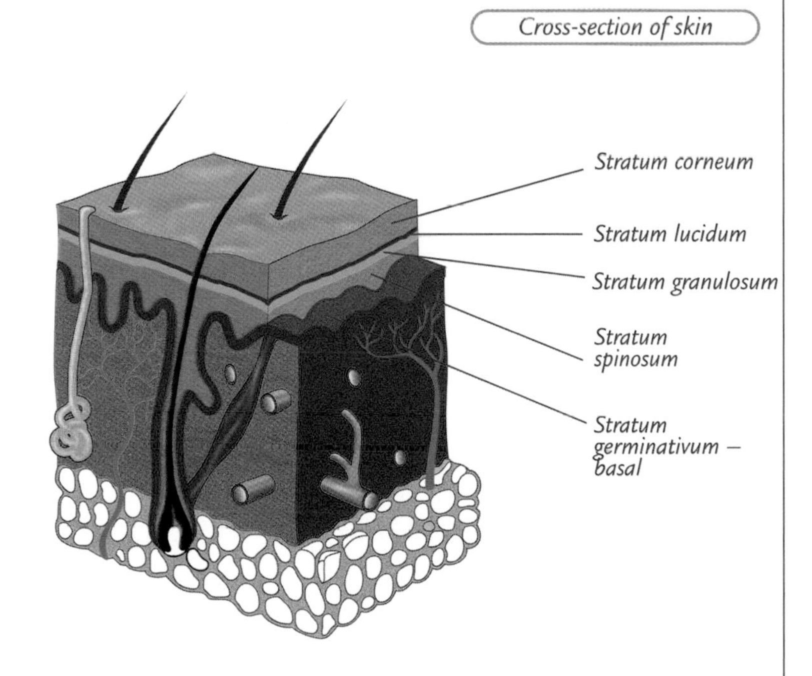

The muscular system

Massage has a direct effect on the muscles. The pumping action helps remove lactic acid, which builds up in overworked or over-exercised muscles, and toxins, thus reducing fatigue and stiffness. Massage improves circulation, which results in quicker delivery of nutrients and oxygen to muscles and faster removal of waste and carbon dioxide which helps muscles to function at their optimum level. Manipulation of muscle leads to relaxation and lengthening of that muscle, improving flexibility and range of movement. Massage also reduces muscle spasms and twitching by reducing the anxiety and tension which causes them.

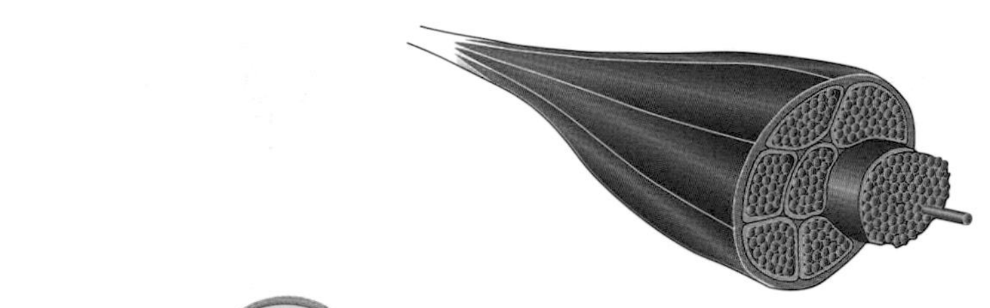

Cross-section of a muscle

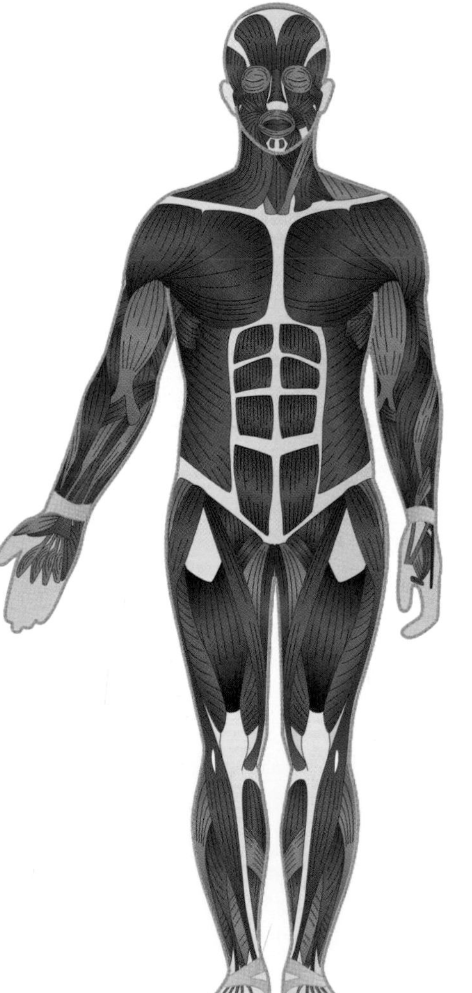

Anterior view of muscles of the body

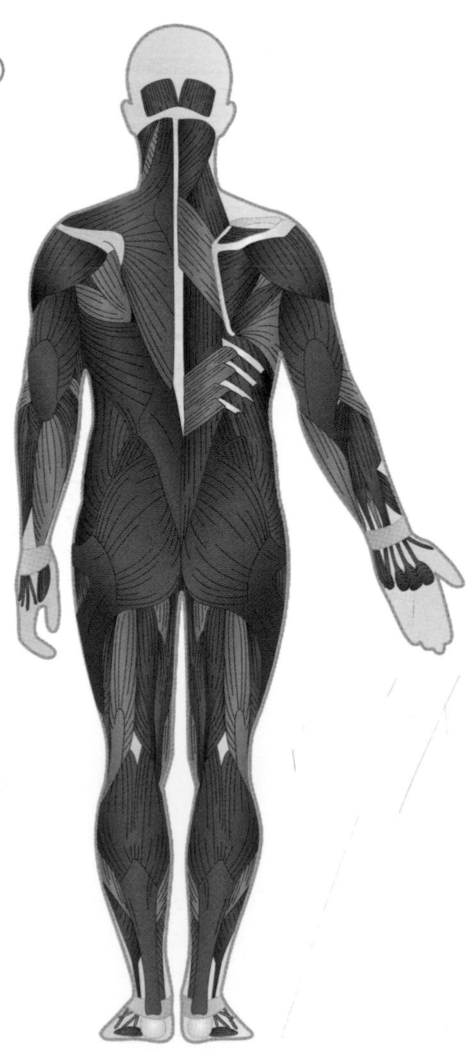

Posterior view of muscles of the body

The circulatory system

Without a continuous blood supply, cells die and the body deteriorates rapidly. The pumping action of massage improves circulation, speeding up the movement of blood in the veins and arteries. Wherever possible the therapist assists the heart by applying pressure towards it. Oxygen and food are delivered more quickly, waste removal is faster and the body therefore functions more efficiently. A gentle massage could lower high blood pressure by reducing the tension which can cause this condition.

The heart

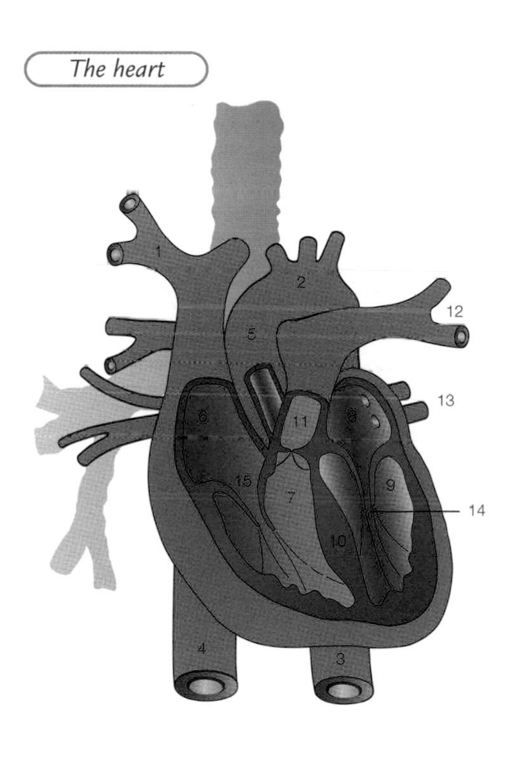

Key

1. *Superior vena cava*
2. *Aortic arch*
3. *Descending aorta*
4. *Inferior vena cava*
5. *Aorta*
6. *Right atrium*
7. *Right ventricle*
8. *Left atrium*
9. *Left ventricle*
10. *Septum*
11. *Pulmonary valve*
12. *Pulmonary arteries*
13. *Pulmonary veins*
14. *Mitral (bicuspid) valve*
15. *Tricuspid valve*

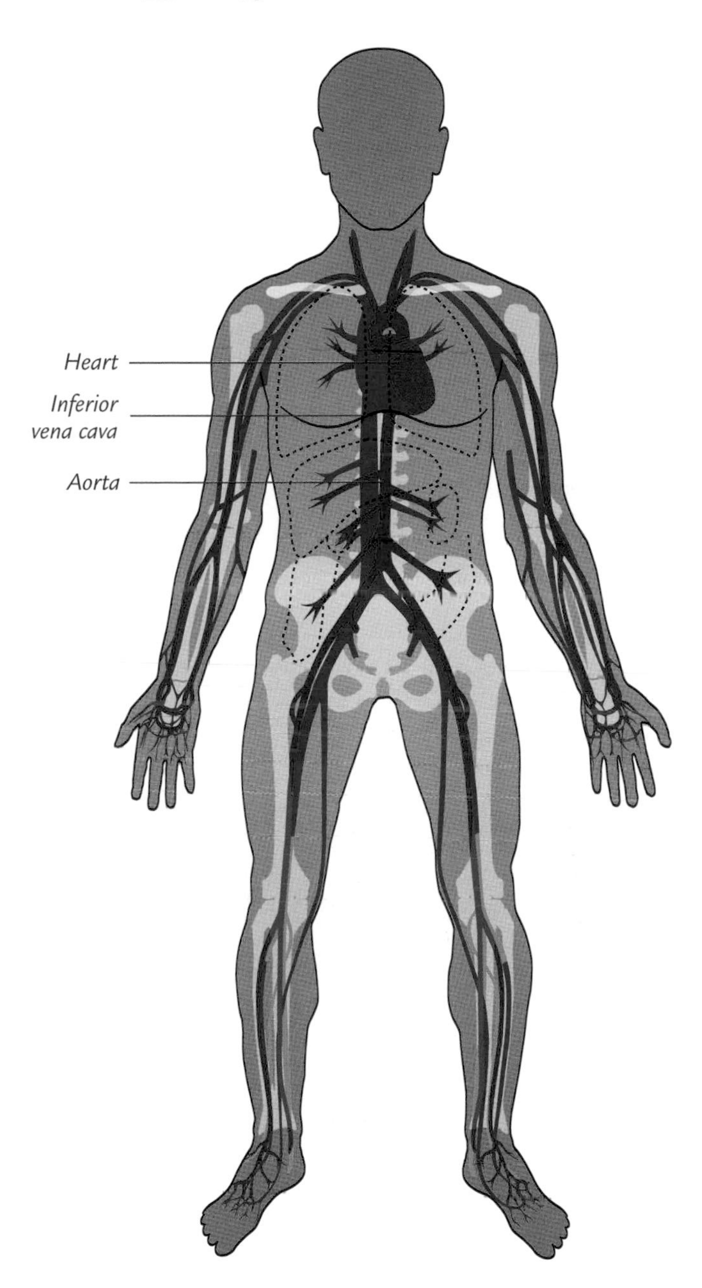

Overview of main arteries and veins

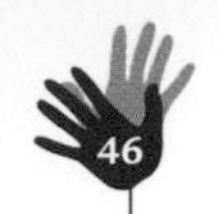

The lymphatic system

Unlike the blood, the lymphatic system has no pump to help it move lymph around the body. Massage is thus very helpful in supporting lymphatic functions, e.g. removal of waste and boosting immunity. It helps reduce swelling (oedema) caused by too much fluid in cells, reduces cellulite and lumpiness and improves lymph circulation. Lymphatic drainage massage, a type of massage used specifically to treat the lymphatic system, is discussed in Chapter 8.

Overview of the lymphatic system showing lymph nodes and spleen

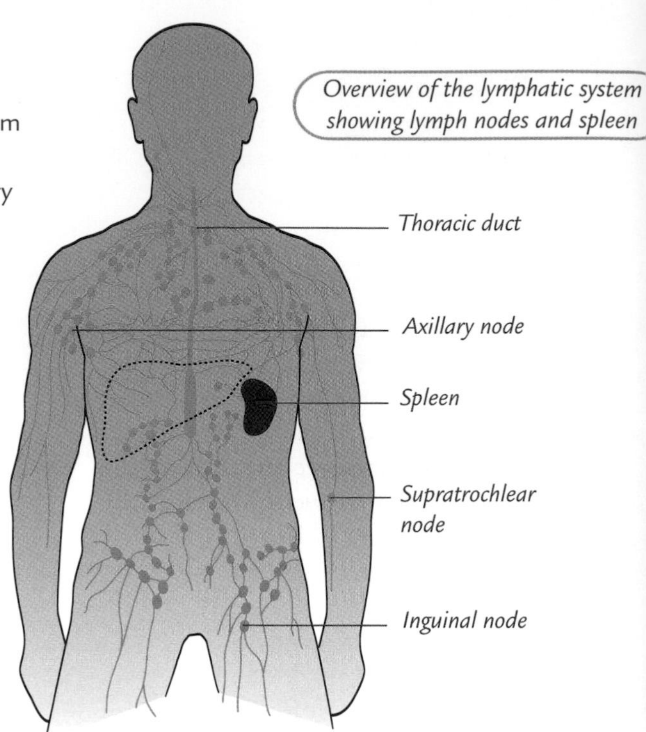

The structure of a nerve cell

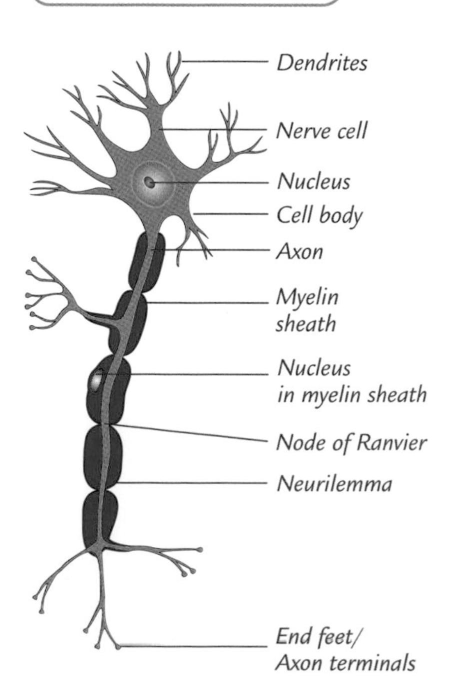

The nervous system

Massage consists of several different techniques, some of which are invigorating whilst others are more relaxing. The effect of a massage on the nervous system will thus depend on the techniques used and the desired goal. For example, a massage to loosen up an athlete before an event is likely to be more stimulating than a massage used to relax a stressed executive. Thus massage can stimulate or relax the nervous system. A massage focused on stimulation will invigorate and wake up the nerves, energising the body. A more relaxing massage will calm the nerves, helping to release tension, stress and promote relaxation.

Other benefits

The following systems all benefit from massage but the effect is more indirect. For example the skeleton will feel less stress because the muscles have been massaged and are working more efficiently.

The skeletal system

The beneficial effects of massage on the muscular system have a positive knock-on effect for the skeleton. The soothing, stroking effleurage techniques of massage help to reduce stiffness and immobility around joints whereas improved muscle flexibility and tone reduces any strain on the joints and bones and improve posture.

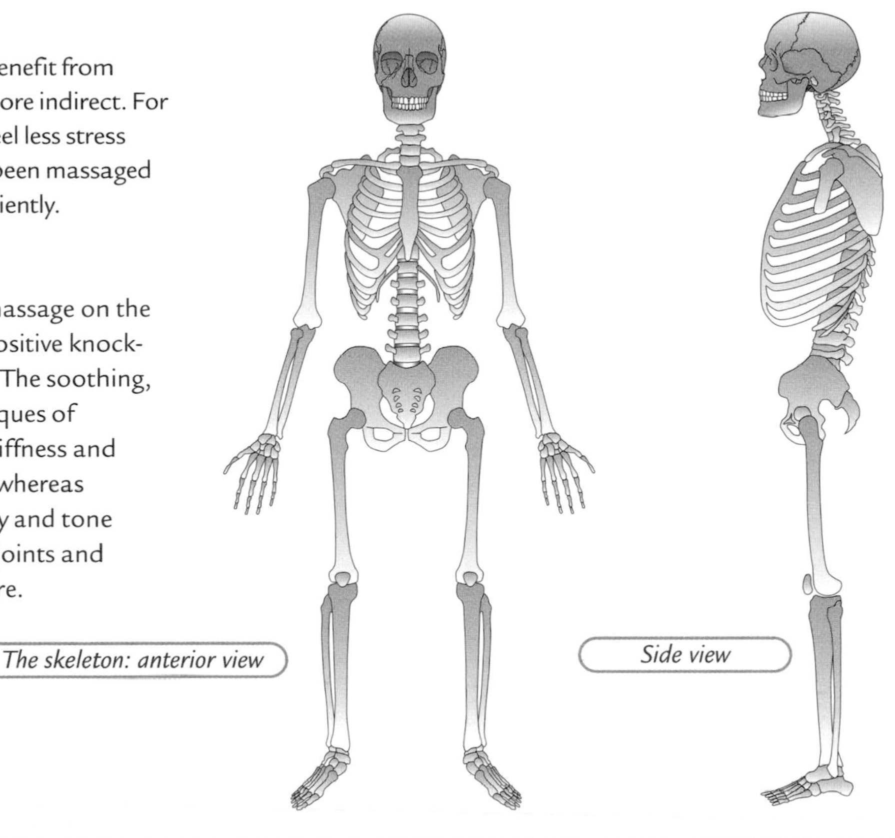

The skeleton: anterior view

Side view

The digestive system

Massage encourages better digestion and assimilation at every level of body function, whether in a cell or in the stomach. It does so by improving the circulation, thus speeding up the delivery of nutrients. It also improves elimination by speeding up the removal of waste and increasing the flow of blood to the liver. Also by improving muscle function it helps strengthen the muscles of the abdomen thus assisting peristalsis and preventing constipation and/or flatulence.

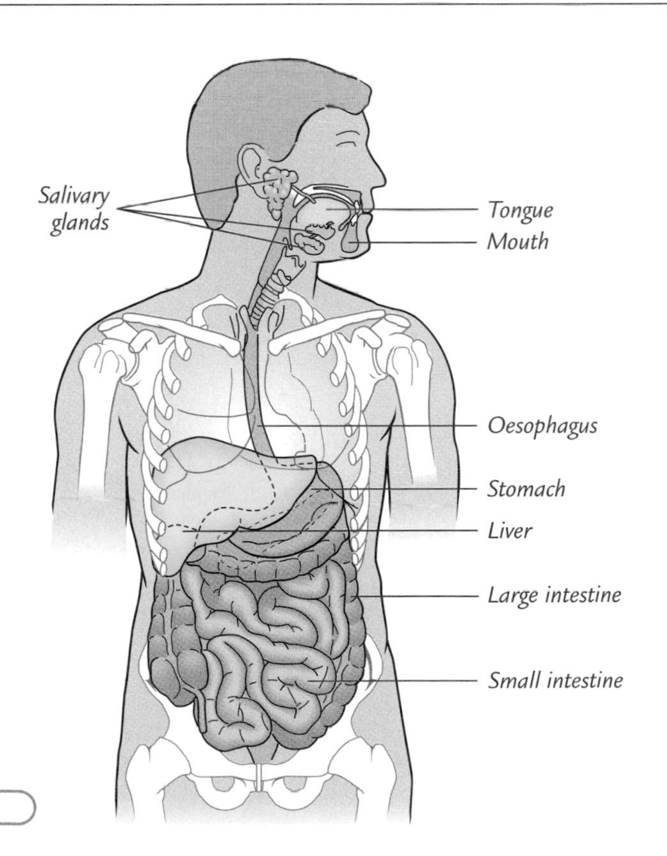

The digestive system

The respiratory system

Massage is very relaxing and when relaxed the body can breathe more easily and deeply. This enables better absorption of oxygen and more efficient removal of carbon dioxide. In addition, the muscles involved in respiration (the diaphragm and intercostal muscles) will be less tense and thus function more efficiently.

The urinary system

Massage encourages better waste removal at every level of body function. It thus encourages urine production and excretion which helps rid the body of toxins and excess liquid.

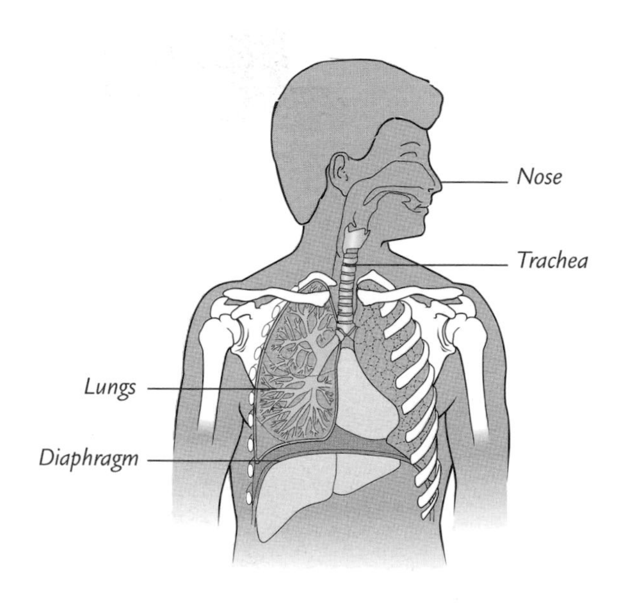

The respiratory system

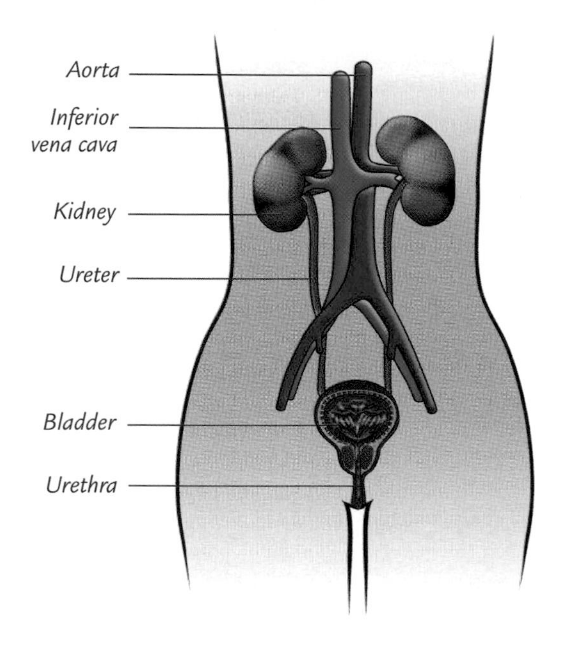

The urinary system (female)

GENERAL SUMMARY

Massage aids circulation, mobilises joints and muscles, improves digestion and by helping overall relaxation, improves and maintains general health.

You now know that massage benefits the whole body and its individual systems.

5 Consultation, treatment & case studies

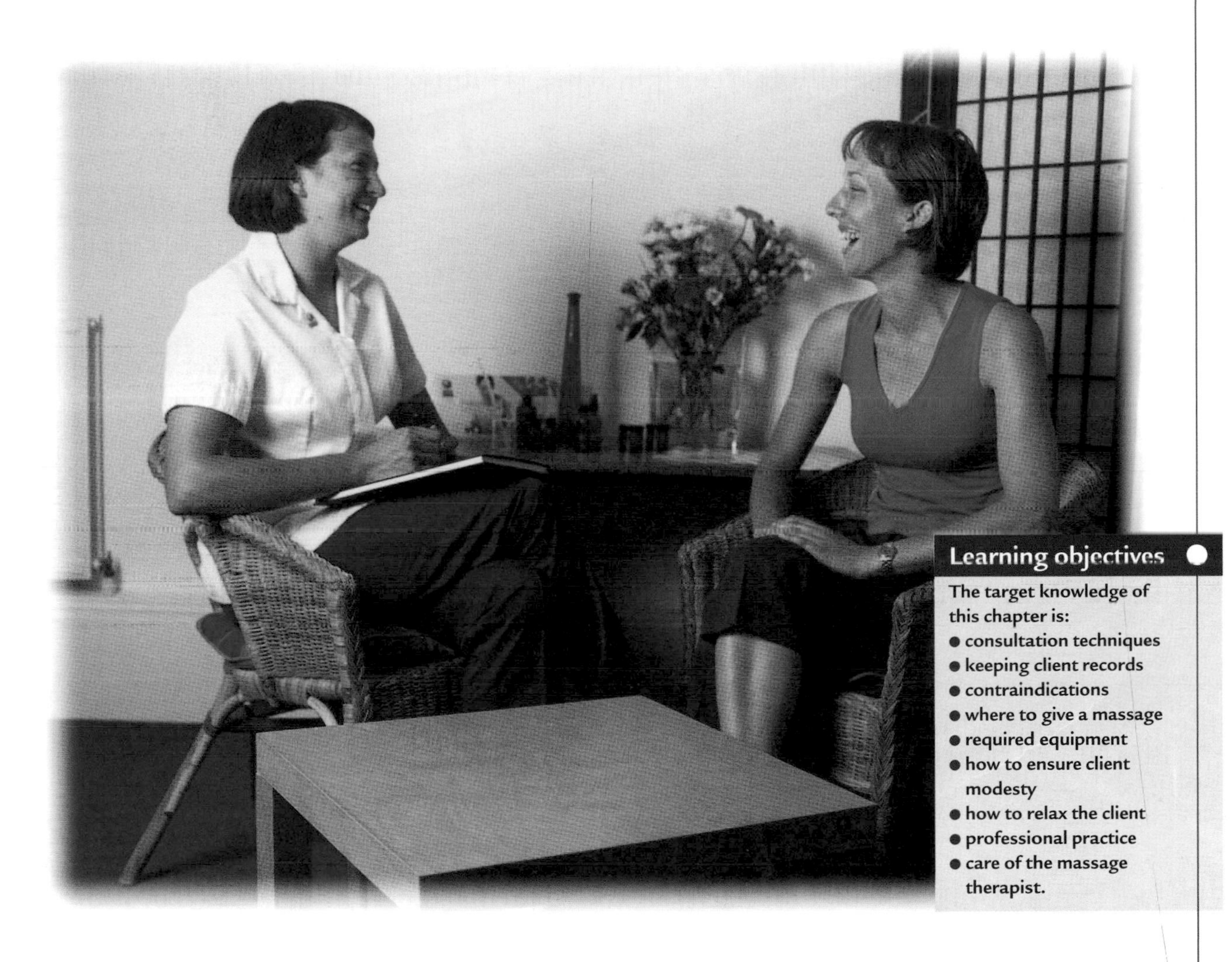

Learning objectives

The target knowledge of this chapter is:

- consultation techniques
- keeping client records
- contraindications
- where to give a massage
- required equipment
- how to ensure client modesty
- how to relax the client
- professional practice
- care of the massage therapist.

In Brief

A massage treatment consists of using massage techniques to promote good health and relaxation. To do this a therapist must know how to find out as much as possible about the client's health and lifestyle so that treatment can be tailored to their requirements. This chapter explains consultation techniques and how to carry out a treatment. It also outlines how the therapist can take care of themself. Throughout this section the person receiving treatment will be referred to as the client.

What is a consultation?

Before treatment can begin the therapist must find out why the client has come for massage and what their expectations are. This is a consultation and it serves as a fact-finding mission for both parties. The therapist must find out about the client's medical history, whether there are any contraindications to treatment and the client's reasons for choosing massage treatment (e.g. is it for a physical problem such as a muscle or joint problem, or poor circulation, for stress or anxiety or simply for relaxation purposes?). The client can find out what the treatment involves and whether it is suitable for their requirements.

As the first contact between therapist and client, the consultation also helps establish a professional relationship. This is especially important with massage treatment because the client must undress and may feel a little uncomfortable about this at the first session. The therapist can reassure the client about any aspect of treatment that concerns them, thus helping an anxious client to relax.

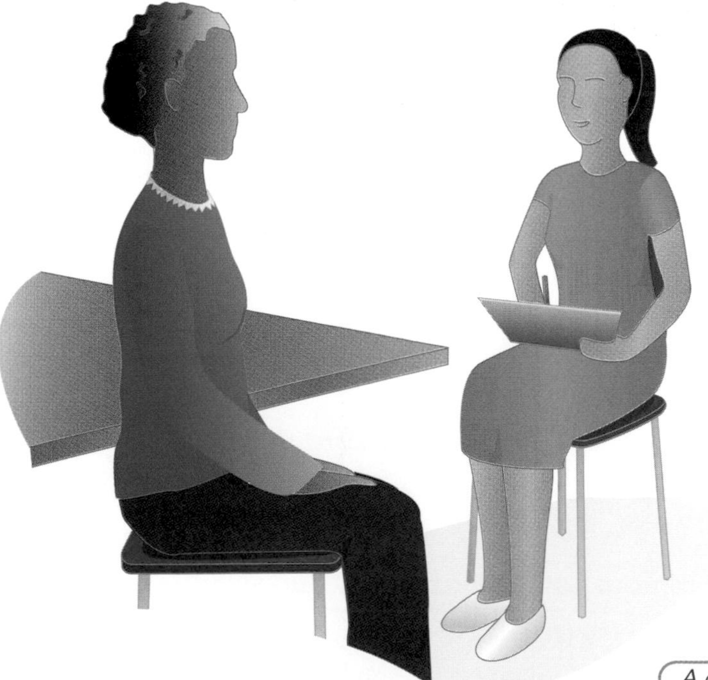

A consultation should cover the following information:

- the client's expectations, and whether these are realistic
- what the treatment involves and the possible effects (i.e. dispelling any unrealistic expectations)
- personal details: name, address, telephone number, date of birth, GP's name and address
- medical background: medicines being taken; medical conditions (any contraindications or problems should be referred; whatever the presenting problem a disclaimer form should be sent to the GP for confirmation that massage will not have any adverse effects); previous illnesses or hereditary diseases; operations; allergies.
- diet and other factors: eating habits, fluid and alcohol consumption, smoker or non-smoker, sleep problems (like insomnia)
- integral biology: work environment, family environment, lifestyle (sedentary or active).

Where do I record the information?

A therapist should keep records of each client's personal details, medical history and treatments. Record-keeping enables a therapist to keep track of a client's progress and the effect of treatment. It is also necessary to prevent abuse of the professional relationship, either by therapist or client. Each therapist will have their own system, e.g. index cards, pre-printed charts or a computer file. Examples of charts are shown opposite. Records should be kept in a locked place to ensure confidentiality. Records kept on a computer must comply with the Data Protection Act.

A consultation taking place

Example of client record

MASSAGE CLIENT RECORD CARD

Client's name: ____________ Date: ____________
Address: ____________ Sex: Male ❑ Female ❑
____________ Date of Birth: ____________
____________ Height: ____________
Tel No: Day: ______ Eve: ______ Weight: ____________
GP Address: ____________ Profession: ____________

Marital Status: Single ❑ Married ❑ Separated ❑ Divorced ❑ Widowed ❑

No. & Age of Children/Dependants: ____________

Pregnant: No ❑ Yes ❑ How many months? ____________

Parental History: ____________

Medical History/Operations: ____________

Medication/Present Health: ____________

Reason for Treatment: ____________

Muscular/Skeletal problems: Neck ❑ Back ❑ Rheumatism ❑ Aches & Pains ❑ Stiff joints ❑ Headaches ❑
Digestive problems: Constipation ❑ Bloating ❑ Liver/gall bladder ❑ Stomach ❑
Circulation: Heart ❑ Blood pressure ❑ Fluid retention ❑ Tired legs ❑ Varicose veins ❑ Cellulite ❑
Kidney problems ❑ Cold hands and feet
Gynaecological: Irregular periods ❑ P.M.T ❑ Menopause ❑ H.R.T ❑ Pill ❑ Coil ❑ Other ____________
Nervous system: Sensitive ❑ Migraine ❑ Tension ❑ Headaches ❑ Stress ❑ Depression ❑
Immune system: Prone to infections ❑ Sore throats ❑ Colds ❑ Chest ❑ Sinuses ❑
Regular antibiotic taken ❑
Professional life (Job details): ____________
Ability to relax: Good ❑ Poor ❑ Average ❑
Time for Self: Hobbies or Creative Interests: ____________
Sleep patterns: Good ❑ Poor ❑ Average no. of hours ❑
Do you see daylight in your workplace? Yes ❑ No ❑
Do you suffer from: Nervous tension ❑ Depression ❑ Anxiety ❑
Do you eat regular meals? Yes ❑ No ❑
Do you eat in a hurry? Yes ❑ No ❑

Do you take food/vitamin supplements? Yes ❑ No ❑
Do you exercise? Yes ❑ No ❑
Is your diet well balanced? Yes ❑ No ❑ ____________
How much of each of these items does your diet contain:
Fresh fruit: ____________
Fresh vegetables: ____________
Protein (source?): ____________
Dairy produce: ____________
Sweet things? ____________
Added salt: ____________ Added sugar: ____________
How many daily drinks of tea: ____________ Coffee: ____________
Fruit Juices: ____________ Water: ____________
Soft Drinks: ____________ Other: ____________
Do you suffer from food allergies? Yes ❑ No ❑ Bingeing: Yes ❑ No ❑ Overeating: Yes ❑ No ❑
Do you smoke? No ❑ Yes ❑ How many per day? __
Do you drink? No ❑ Light ❑ Medium ❑ Heavy ❑ Units per week: ____________
Do you exercise? None ❑ Occasional ❑ Irregular ❑ Regular ❑ Types: ____________
What is your skin type: Dry ❑ Oily ❑ Combination ❑ Sensitive ❑ Dehydrated ❑
Do you suffer from: Dermatitis: Yes ❑ No ❑ Acne: Yes ❑ No ❑ Eczema: Yes ❑ No ❑
Psoriasis: Yes ❑ No ❑ Allergies: Yes ❑ No ❑ Hay Fever: Yes ❑ No ❑ Asthma: Yes ❑ No ❑

Client's Signature: ____________

Treatment results

Treatment 1

Treatment 2

Treatment 3

Treatment 4

Overall conclusion

What are the contraindications to massage?

Massage is non-invasive, relaxing and natural. It is therefore generally considered a safe treatment for most people. However, there are three types of contraindication: total, when massage should not be performed at all, localised, when massage can be performed over the rest of the body but not over the contraindicated areas; medical, when massage can only be performed once medical permission has been granted.

Total contraindications

When a client has any of these conditions the therapist should not massage:

- fever
- contagious or infectious diseases
- under the influence of drugs or alcohol
- cancer (unless in terminal stages and then with medical permission).

Local

The therapist can massage but not over any areas affected by:

- skin diseases
- undiagnosed lumps or bumps
- varicose veins
- pregnancy (on the abdomen, with medical permission)
- cuts
- bruises
- abrasions
- inflammation
- scar tissue (two years for major operation and six months for a small scar)
- sunburn
- areas of undiagnosed pain
- menstruation – on the abdomen, for the first few days or depending on how the client is feeling.

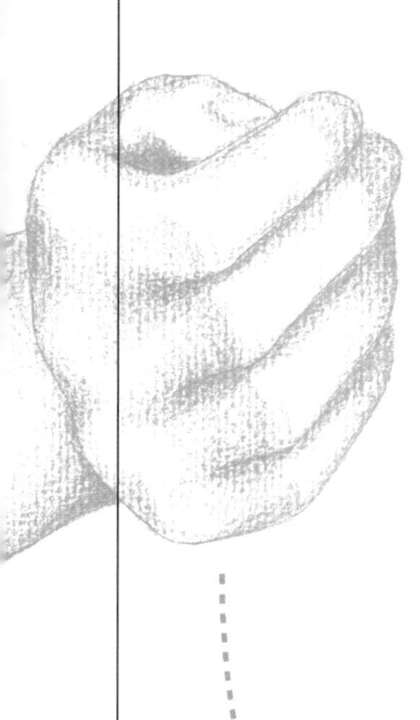

Medical

If the client suffers from any of the following conditions, massage can only take place once it has been approved by a GP:

- pregnancy
- cardio-vascular conditions (thrombosis, phlebitis, hypertension, hypotension, heart conditions)
- any condition already being treated by a GP or another complementary therapy practitioner
- medical oedema
- osteoporosis
- arthritis
- nervous/psychotic conditions
- epilepsy
- recent operations
- diabetes
- asthma
- Bell's palsy
- trapped or pinched nerves
- inflamed nerve
- acute rheumatism.

Does a contraindication mean that treatment cannot take place?

Not always. However, in the above cases and whenever you are unsure whether it is safe to proceed, it is best to refer the client to their GP for advice. The therapist should not, under any circumstances, attempt to diagnose a condition or decide whether an existing condition is treatable. The code of conduct of many complementary health associations states that diagnosis is not allowed. If there is any uncertainty, refer the client.

How and where do I carry out a consultation?

A consultation should take place in a comfortable, private room, where there is no chance of interruption. The room can be used for both consultation and treatment as long as it is possible to do so in a relaxed manner, i.e. do not sit behind a desk, and try to project an open, friendly image – keep arms and legs uncrossed, establish eye contact and smile. The client must feel reassured and comfortable in order to answer the questions and also to fully benefit from

the treatment. Finally, the consultation should always take place when the client is fully dressed, not only because it prevents them feeling embarrassed or vulnerable, but also because it prevents the therapist feeling awkward if the treatment is contraindicated for the client and cannot take place. The consultation form should be re-checked at every appointment.

First impressions

Everything the therapist does communicates a message to the client and can affect the treatment. First impressions are very important, especially the first touch. If you choose to greet a client with a handshake remember that this is the first time you will touch them. A handshake that is limp, damp, sweaty, too firm or too weak may communicate to the client, either consciously or unconsciously, that the massage will have the same qualities. This could make them anxious or tense if they disliked the feeling. Be aware of this and act accordingly. Practice with friends to make sure that your handshake is relaxed and confident. If you have a tendency to sweaty palms use a light dusting of talc to counteract this. The first touch when beginning a massage is equally important: it needs to be firm, relaxed and smooth not ticklish, tentative or damp.

How do I get information from my client?

A new client may feel a little uneasy or nervous about the treatment, about being semi-undressed in front of a stranger or about revealing information about themselves. So your first task is to reassure and relax them by explaining what the treatment involves, how client modesty will be maintained through the use of towels and how all information will help you tailor treatment to their needs. You must also stress that all records are confidential. The next step is to encourage them to volunteer the required information. You will soon be able to judge how to approach this with different clients. For example, an open and relaxed person will need little coaxing but with shy, reticent clients a therapist will need to demonstrate listening skills. The following list of suggestions will help you get the most from a consultation.

- Start with general questions or, if you want to prompt , or sense a particularly shy client, use the form/record card as a starting point. Once you have begun asking questions which are easy to answer (name, address, date of birth etc) the more difficult ones about treatment and contraindications won't seem so daunting — the client will be in the rhythm of responding to your questions and will expect them rather than be made more nervous.
- Ask open not closed questions - ones that cannot be answered with yes or no. For example, ask 'What do you expect from a massage?' rather than 'Do you expect the massage to work?' or 'Tell me about your diet' rather than 'Do you eat healthily?'. No one likes to examine their own habits so it is best to address the questions in as open and unthreatening manner as possible.
- In order to instil trust, use your own body language to encourage and aid responses: nodding, smiling and leaning forward all communicate interest as does keeping eye contact. Looking away frequently, fidgeting or staring blankly will merely communicate nervousness and/or lack of interest, which will not help the

client to feel confident in your abilities or your interest in them. Remember that, as a therapist, you are there to help the client. If you are unfriendly, nervous or uncommunicative the client is likely to pick up on this and react in a similar way.

- Be confident, enthusiastic and professional.
- Communicate your own belief and trust in the treatment – this will help the client to believe in it and will improve the psychological and physiological effects of the massage.
- Reassure the client that everything discussed will remain completely confidential and make sure that you never break this confidence.
- Treat everyone equally. If you cannot avoid bringing racist or sexist prejudices to the massage table then this is not the profession for you.

You now know how to carry out a consultation and find out the information needed to give an effective and safe massage. The next section explains how to carry out a treatment.

HOW TO CARRY OUT A TREATMENT

Where should a massage be given?

Massage requires the client to be partly or completely undressed (underpants should be kept on). The treatment room should therefore be private and without risk of interruption. Fear of someone entering the room will usually cause the client to tense up thus preventing or counteracting the positive, relaxing benefits of the massage. The room should have enough space for both the couch and the therapist to move around it and work. It should also be the correct temperature, i.e. not too cold or too warm. You will be much warmer than the client because you will be exerting yourself physically. Make sure that there is a suitable ambient temperature. Towels should be neatly placed under and over the client, covering up any area of the body which is not currently being massaged. A blanket may be used on top of the towels at the beginning of the massage or during it, as necessary, to keep the client warm. The lighting in the room should be indirect and conducive to relaxation but bright enough to allow the therapist to work. Lamps with adjustable angles and brightness are preferable to glaring, overhead lighting.

What equipment is needed?

1) a massage couch

To perform a massage comfortably and effectively a height-adjustable couch covered with towels is recommended. Couch roll (disposable paper that can be pulled over the couch/towels) can be used to prevent the towels being stained by massage oil. If couch roll has not been used, the towels must be changed for each client. The couch should be firmly padded, to prevent the pressure of the massage being absorbed by soft cushioning under the body, easy to clean and wide and long enough to accommodate different clients. Some couches have a face hole, with a flap, to enable a client's head and spine to remain aligned when face down, but not all clients will require this or like it. Remember that the therapist should also be comfortable and not straining or overstretching to perform the treatment. A couch that can be adjusted to the right height for each individual prevents such problems. The couch should be at the therapist's hip height and the therapist should be able to extend an arm and comfortably place a hand, palm down, flat on the couch.

See also the 'Care of the therapist' section at the end of this chapter.

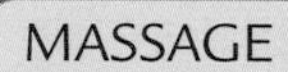

2) pillows and towels for support and protection
Pillows will help both client and therapist. For a massage on the back, pillows or rolled towels under the shoulders and ankles will help improve comfort. Using a face hole in the couch will help keep the head and spine properly aligned during a back massage. (However, not all clients will be comfortable using one.) Additionally, a pillow can be used under the chest for client comfort. For a front of the body massage a pillow under the neck and under the knees will provide support, relax the back and prevent strain. As mentioned earlier, towels are required to cover the parts of the client which are not being massaged.

3) couch roll (disposable paper)
Couch roll is optional. It can be used to protect towels from being stained by massage or essential oil.

4) changing facilities and bathroom
The client should be able to undress in privacy so adequate changing facilities will be required. Most local authorities also require that a shower should be available for client use. A large towel or robe should be provided for the client to wrap themselves in after undressing. Underpants should be kept on and spectacles/contact lenses and jewellery removed. It is advisable that both therapist and client go to the toilet before the massage begins to prevent interruption.

5) trolley
One or both hands should always be kept on the body being massaged during the treatment, since as soon as the hands are removed, the body registers this as the end of the massage and begin to 'change gear', waking up from the relaxation. Any form of interruption will disrupt the massage and lessen its positive effects. However, during the massage the therapist may need to reach the oil, cream or talc being used or extra towels. Ready-wipes or cotton wool and surgical spirit should also be available. A trolley stocked with the required equipment and moved around the room to convenient positions prevents unnecessary interruptions.

How do I ensure client modesty?
For most massage treatments, the client will need to undress to their underpants. A large towel or robe should be provided in the changing facilities for the client to wrap themselves in after undressing. Once on the couch, this large towel can be used to cover the upper body at the beginning and end of the massage. A second towel is used to cover the lower body. During treatment towels should be draped over the client, covering up any area of the

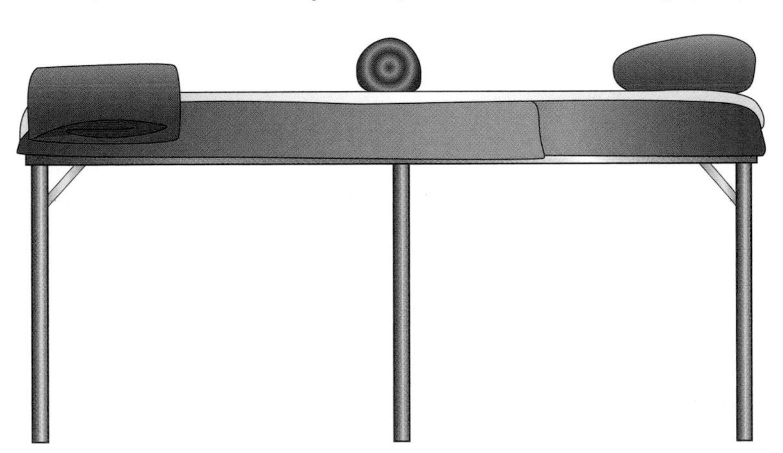

A couch set up for massage

body which is not currently being massaged. The towels help keep the client warm as well as ensuring that they do not feel exposed. At the end of the treatment the large towel can once again be used as a wrap for the body and the therapist should help the client off the couch so that they can hold on to the wrap.

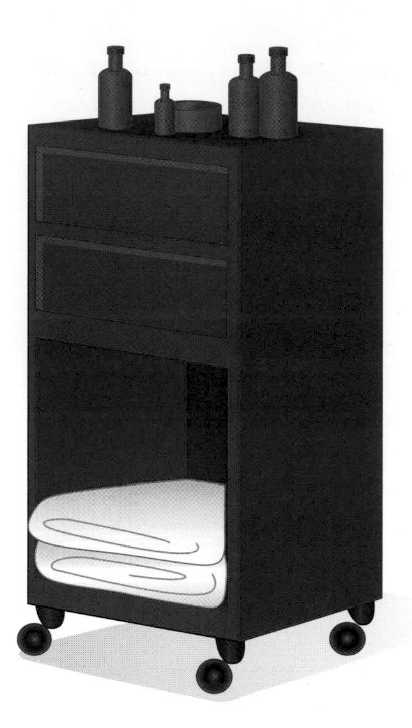

Trolley set up for use during treatment

How do I make sure the client can relax?

Hopefully, the client will feel more relaxed after the consultation. However, there are several other factors which can help. As discussed earlier, the room should be a comfortable temperature, the client's privacy should never be compromised and lighting should be bright enough for the massage to be carried out but not harsh. In addition, to make the treatment as comfortable and secure as possible there should be no chance of interruption; windows should be shielded with blinds or curtains; changing facilities should open into the treatment room or be positioned as close as possible so that the client does not have to walk very far once undressed. A footstool or step may be placed by the couch to enable the client to get onto the couch without immodesty (this is especially useful for elderly, shorter or less flexible clients). Once installed on the couch check that they are comfortable and warm enough. Ask if they wish to listen to music and if so play something quiet and soothing rather than loud and upbeat. Some clients may prefer to talk, some may prefer silence. Remember that this is their time and you should respect their wishes – they are not paying to hear your views or personal

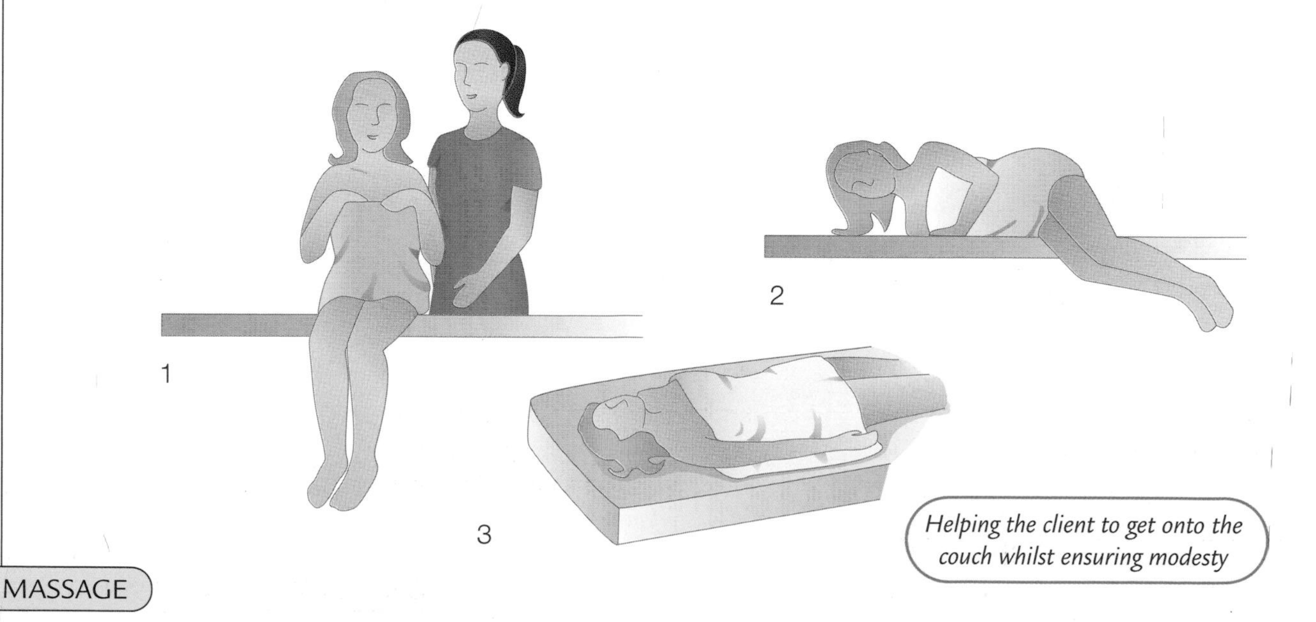

Helping the client to get onto the couch whilst ensuring modesty

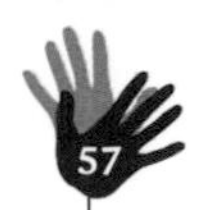

preferences. During the massage listen to their comments, if any, and adjust the treatment accordingly, adding or reducing pressure or work on a particular area if necessary.

What happens at the end of the massage?

Throughout the treatment you will have been using oil, cream or talc. At the end this needs to be removed from the skin. Most clients will simply choose to shower and wash off the medium. However, if for any reason this is not possible (because the client prefers not to shower rather than the shower not being available, which may contravene local authority regulations) or desirable, damp cotton wool should be used to remove the medium, followed by a skin toner and/or a hot towel.

Once this is completed, re-cover the whole body with the large towel and discreetly help the client to wrap themselves in it.When they are sitting up, help them off the couch. Once the client has dressed let them sit still for a moment, to give them time to 'wake up'. You may like to offer them a glass of water because massage often causes thirstiness, and water will help flush out released toxins.

Aftercare advice

After treatment many reactions can be experienced. You should explain to the client that this is a positive result of the treatment. Massage makes the body systems function more efficiently, speeding up waste removal and the elimination of toxins. Thus the after-effects may include:

- frequent urination
- headaches
- thirst
- sleepiness.

Good professional practice

It is extremely important for any therapist to take the following information into consideration when performing a massage.

- **emotions and sex**

When carrying out a massage it is evident that the client will be semi-naked. His or her modesty is of paramount importance and a professional therapist will not allow any emotional or sexual involvement with the client to compromise the client's position. Vice-versa, if you feel that the client is behaving inappropriately towards you, you would be perfectly within your rights to discontinue the treatment.

- **psychology**

It is important not to become the client's counsellor. Obviously, if a client feels relaxed and comfortable with the therapist, he or she may discuss their personal matters but the therapist must resist the temptation to get involved, offering judgements or advice. It is also wise to avoid topics of conversation that may cause offence or strong feelings such as money, marriage, religion or politics.

- **hygiene**

The equipment (couch, towels, changing room and consultation room) should be kept clean at all times and the therapist should also pay attention to his or her personal hygiene since they will be spending intensive periods of time in a confined space with the client. Good hygiene is essential for ensuring a professional image and protecting the health of both therapist and client.

- **professional image**

The person giving the massage should be dressed comfortably in professional clothes and comfortable, flat shoes. Nails should be kept short, clean and

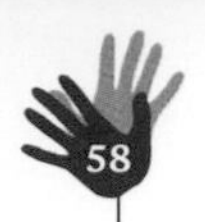

unvarnished and jewellery avoided. Where necessary, hair should be pinned or tied away from the face and off the collar.

You now know how to set up an area for giving a massage, how to ensure the client feels relaxed and comfortable and what constitutes good professional practice. The next section explains how the massage therapist can protect themselves whilst working.

CARE OF THE MASSAGE THERAPIST

As you can probably tell from Chapter 3, massage is a very physical treatment. The effects of this treatment depend on the physical energy of the therapist performing it. If, for any reason, that energy is depleted by health problems or limited by incorrect posture then the treatment will be less effective. Furthermore, any therapist continuing to work without paying attention to posture and correct working positions will cause damage to their own body, both in the short- and long-term. This section explains how massage therapists can take care of themselves, both in preparation for working and during treatment, in order to protect their health and carry out effective massages.

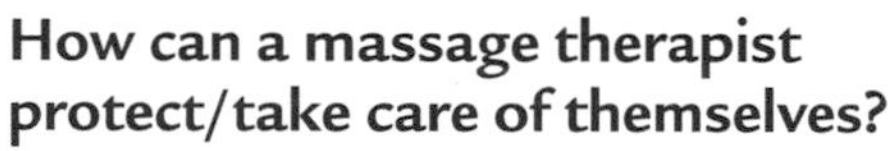

How can a massage therapist protect/take care of themselves?

In order to protect themselves, massage therapists should pay attention to the following four areas: posture, working position, attitude and exercise. Each one of these factors contributes to the positive effects of treatment and prevents the therapist from damaging themselves.

What is posture?

Posture is the way we position and hold our body.

How can it help the massage therapist?

Good posture is necessary both professionally and physically. When greeting and treating clients, a therapist must always be aware of how they are holding themselves. This is both protective and demonstrative: many clients will have back and joint problems caused by incorrect posture and if the therapist is explaining how poor posture can cause these problems it helps if they themselves are following such advice.

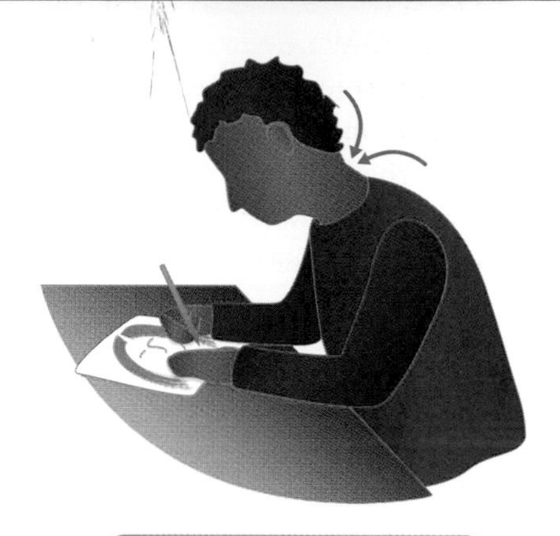

Incorrect sitting posture

When consulting and working the therapist should avoid:

- tension in arms, neck and shoulders
- stiff, rigid legs and locked knees
- stiff, inflexible wrists and hands
- uneven distribution of weight in the legs, i.e. resting on one more than the other
- bending without using the knees
- bending the spine
- slouching or crossing the legs whilst consulting
- repeating the same movements: varying the routines helps prevent repetitive strain injuries
- overstretching across the couch.

All of the above can cause back and neck problems, muscle strain and repetitive strain injuries. Not only are they damaging, they also affect the therapist's attitude (see below), give a poor impression and prevent the most effective treatment.

What is the correct posture for massage treatment?

There is no absolutely correct posture because everyone's body is different. However, a therapist should:

- keep the back straight but not rigid
- keep wrists and forearms as straight as possible without locking them
- keep legs slightly bent
- keep shoulders relaxed; it is a common tendency to tense shoulders, holding them close to the ears. Practice rolling them away from the ears and towards the ground in order to release this.
- move around the couch instead of overreaching and risking muscle damage.
- distribute the weight of the body evenly between both legs. Many of us tend to rest on one leg, overworking it and weakening the other.
- take regular breaks (though not, of course, during a treatment).
- use a height-adjustable couch positioned so that it is possible to extend the arms and place the palms of the hands flat on the surface of the couch without strain.
- be aware of their own body, where tension is held and what causes strain. Awareness of one's own body's limits will help prevent overstretching it.
- remember that it is often the tiniest movements which cause the most damage.

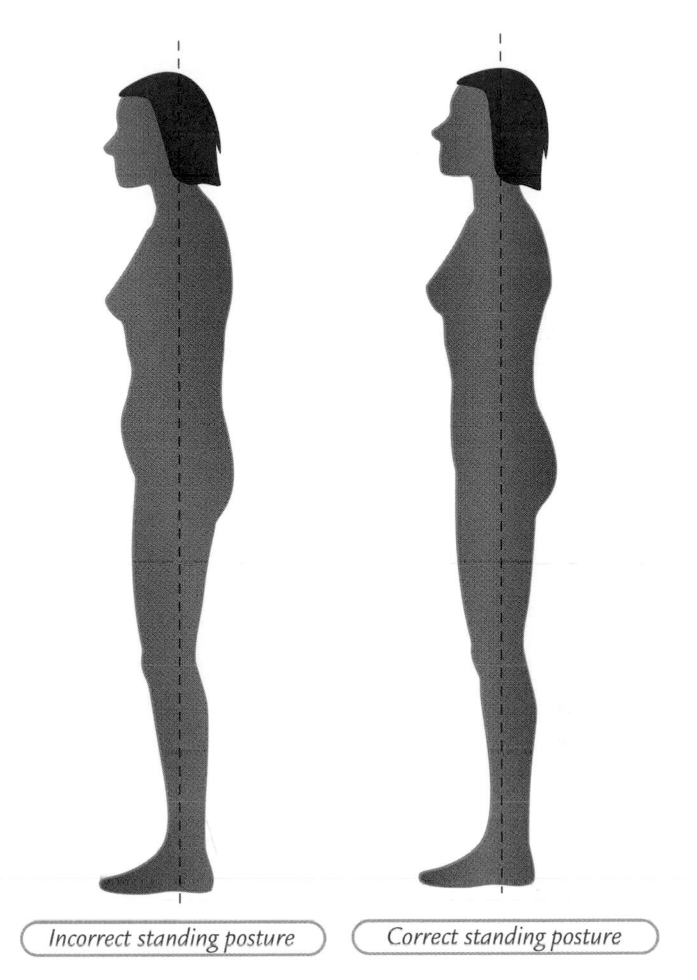

Incorrect standing posture | *Correct standing posture*

Why is correct posture important to the treatment?

Massage is a very physical treatment and correct posture helps the therapist perform to the best of their abilities without damaging themselves. If the therapist is evenly balanced, with weight evenly distributed through the legs and pelvis, flexible and relaxed, the massage will be smooth, rhythmic and relaxed. If the therapist is moving in a jerky or unbalanced way, often as a result of tension in the body or an uneven distribution of weight in the legs, the treatment will also be jerky. Furthermore, good posture enables the therapist to concentrate on the massage without worrying about their own body and whether they will be able to perform the movements.

You now know why good posture is important to a massage therapist.

WORKING POSITION

What is a working position?

A working position is a stance adopted by the therapist whilst carrying out a treatment.

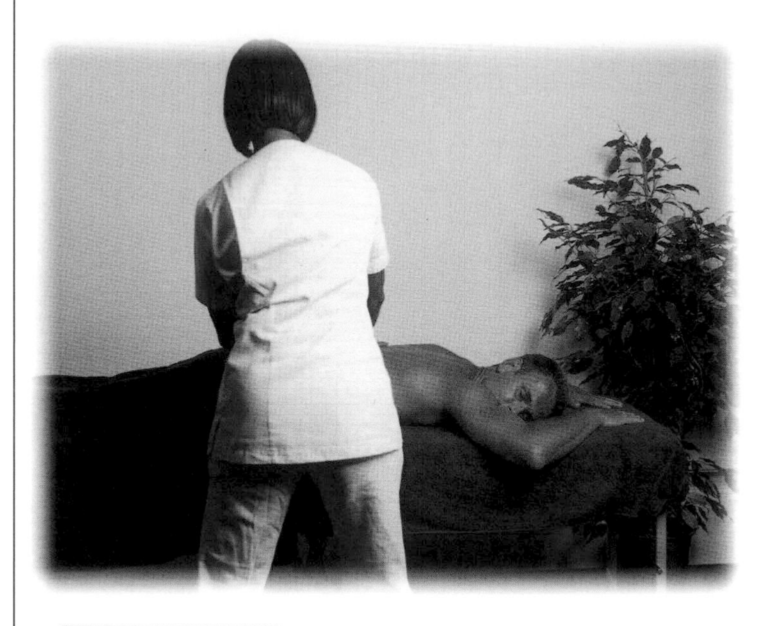

Side standing position

How does it help the therapist?

Working positions are designed to protect the working therapist from muscle or joint strain as well as allow maximum mobility and pressure for the treatment. The following working positions are recommended for full body massage.

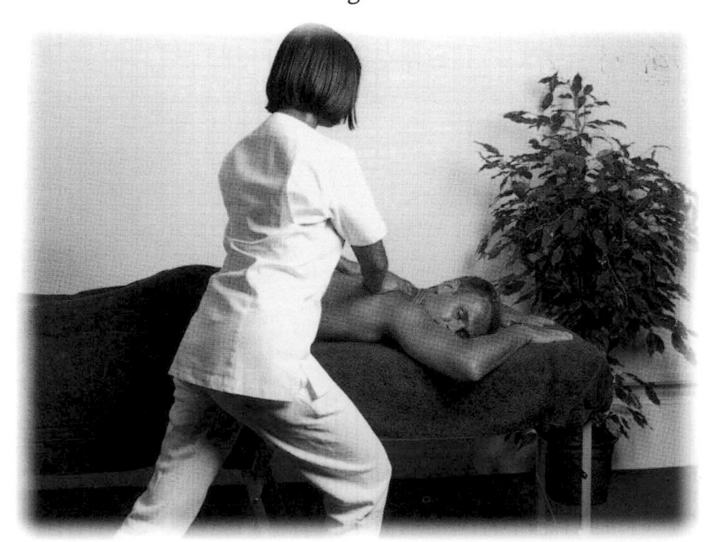

- **Side standing position**

Place feet approximately 30cm apart with toes just under and in line with the edge of the couch and pointing out at 45 degrees, knees soft, hips forward, bottom tucked under, forearms at right angles to the body with wrists kept in alignment with arms and flexible. Be careful not to stiffen shoulders, knees or lower back and not to hang the head in order to look down. Keep the neck straight and look down from this position or, if this is not possible, tilt the head slightly by lowering the jaw rather than bending the neck. You can also have a wider stance and bend the knees more, to get closer to your client. This position is used for short strokes, such as petrissage and percussion, rather than effleurage, when work is across the muscles or on a local area not a whole section.

- **Striding position**

Stand with the body at an angle to the table, feet positioned as if striding forward, one in front of the other. The knees need to be flexible not rigid and it is important to bend from the waist and not from the middle of the back. This position is used for strokes along the length of the body particularly the back and limbs. The therapist uses the striding position to push themselves forwards along the body. The weight is moved from the back foot to the front foot and this gives momentum to the stroke, as if the movement that the therapist should be making, given the position of the feet, is transmitted to the arms.

You now know how to position yourself when working.

Striding position

ATTITUDE

What is attitude?

Attitude is the mental equivalent of posture. It is the disposition of the mind, how someone is thinking and feeling. Someone with a positive attitude is thinking and feeling positive.

Why is it important for the massage therapist?

Have you ever noticed that when you're in a good mood and you meet someone in a bad or negative mood, you often leave them feeling much less positive? This is because we are affected by other people's emotional moods and attitudes. When carrying out a massage a therapist's mood and attitude will affect their client. So a tense therapist will make the client tense, a hurried therapist will make the client feel rushed. A tense or hurried therapist is also more likely to damage themselves whilst working. If the massage is to have the desired effect, whether relaxing or energising, the therapist will need the right attitude. In general, the therapist should feel centred and focused, secure and calm and able to concentrate on using their own physical or mental energy to work on and improve the physical and mental energy of the client. Yoga, meditation and t'ai chi are all exercises for the mind and body which are useful for concentration and focus.

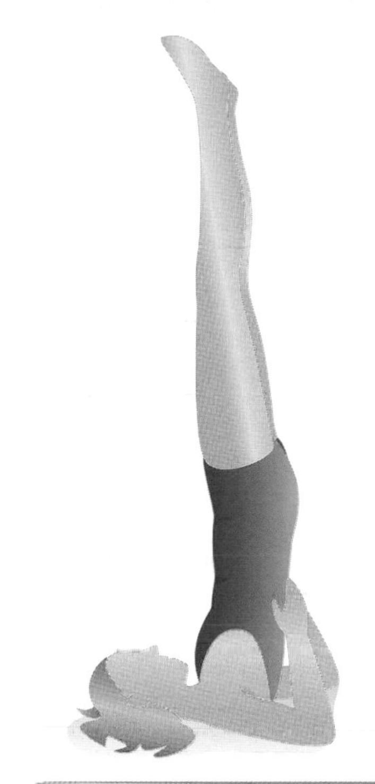

Yoga posture – a shoulder stand

Exercise and breathing

A massage therapist will need to take regular exercise in order to have the physical fitness and stamina to carry out treatment. Exercise is also one of the best ways to relax after work, in order to prevent the build-up of tension and stiffness from working in similar standing positions all day. Hands and wrists should also be exercised on a regular basis to keep them supple and flexible. Finally, breathing exercises can help with relaxation both during and between treatments. Throughout the massage the therapist should be aware of their breathing and that of the client. They should encourage the client to breathe deeply and evenly and should make sure their own breathing is calm, regular and matches the client's pace. This will enable both parties to relax and concentrate on the treatment. Relaxation and breathing techniques are part of yoga, meditation and t'ai chi. It can be very beneficial for a massage therapist to themselves receive regular massage therapy.

You now know how to consult with a client and how to look after yourself as the therapist.

SWEDISH MASSAGE

Client profile

John is a 26-year-old computer consultant. He spends a lot of time using a computer, both at work and at home, and as a result suffers from back and shoulder ache. He does not exercise, drinks and smokes on a daily basis and is not on any medication. He came for massage to relieve his stiff back and shoulders.

Summary of treatment

John had four full-body Swedish massage treatments over the space of four weeks.

Week 1: The massage started with plenty of effleurage all over the back for relaxation and getting him used to the touch. The massage then concentrated on kneading up the latissimus dorsi and around the trapezius muscles, petrissage up the erector spinae and working around the scapula, particularly the rhomboid muscles, with thumb frictions After this treatment he was surprised to feel extremely tired and very thirsty. He was advised that this was a natural part of the healing process and that one way of preventing dehydration is to drink plenty of water, both immediately after treatment and in the following days.

Week 2: The day after the massage John commented that he felt very tired and ached quite a bit in his back but after 48 hours his back was feeling much better. There did not appear to be so much tension in the muscles but there was still quite a bit in the trapezius muscle, particularly across the shoulders. Kneading and petrissage were used to try to release the lactic acid around these areas.

Week 3: It again took John about two days for his back to feel better. He found the aftercare advice of drinking plenty of water useful, along with getting up from the computer every half hour and exercising his arms and shoulders to keep his back from stiffening. Again the massage concentrated on kneading and petrissage around the trapezius but also plenty of petrissage along the erector spinae. His back felt much more pliable and he appeared to be standing more upright and looking much more relaxed.

Week 4: John commented that he had not felt as much pain during the first 24 hours as he had previously and agreed that the massage sessions had really helped. A normal back massage was given this session using all the movements. John's shoulders and upper back were much looser and less painful. He had decided to do more exercise and felt that this, along with the massage, was improving his energy levels.

AROMATHERAPY MASSAGE

Client profile

Rachel is a 40-year-old nightclub manager. She works nights and finds this very stressful and disruptive. She also lives alone and finds this depressing, especially since she would like to settle down and have children. She does little exercise, does not drink but smokes 20 cigarettes per day. She is not on any medication. She wanted aromatherapy massage to lift her spirits and relieve some of her stress.

Summary of treatment

Rachel had four full-body aromatherapy massages over the space of four weeks.

Week 1: In the first treatment sweet orange, neroli and frankincense essential oils were used in a blend with peach kernel oil. Sweet orange is anti-depressant, neroli soothes the nerves and frankincense is calming. Rachel found it relaxing as well as cheering, the citrus scent dispelling the gloomy weather which was depressing her.

Week 2: After a hectic and unbalanced week, Rachel felt that she needed some balance. Lavender, geranium and bergamot essential oils were used in a blend with peach kernel oil. Lavender and geranium are both balancing oils whereas bergamot, a member of the citrus family, is uplifting. Rachel found the treatment very calming and she said that after the massage she slept better than she had done for months. Also, as a result of her improved mood she has found time in the day to get out for a walk and has found that the exercise is giving her more energy.

Week 3: Rachel's enthusiasm indicated another uplifting blend: grapefruit, bergamot and lavender. She reported that after the massage, when she went straight to work she had felt more able to cope with her job and the stress involved. In week four the weather became much warmer and this, combined with the treatment, made Rachel feel more positive and calm.

Week 4: The final massage used a blend of rosemary, cypress and sweet orange essential oils with apricot kernel oil as the carrier. Rosemary is calming, cypress is a tonic and sweet orange is antidepressant. Rachel has decided to continue with massage treatment to help maintain her positive attitude.

ON-SITE MASSAGE

Client profile

Maureen is a 55-year-old divorcee with two children, one of whom lives at home. She is generally a very relaxed person but the combination of a full-time job, financial worries and looking after her 16 year old son is starting to cause her high levels of stress, resulting in many headaches. She wanted a massage to help her relax but didn't want it at home as her son would comment about the expense so with her boss's approval she had an on-site massage at her desk during her lunch break. Maureen walks to work every day, drinks socially and does not smoke. She is not on any medication.

Summary of treatment

Maureen had four 15-minute head, neck and shoulder massages over four weeks.

Week 1: The massage was concentrated around the deltoid, upper trapezius, neck and head areas. Effleurage was performed all over to help relax the client and get her used to the pressure. Maureen preferred quite a deep pressure so kneading and petrissage were used initially, particularly up the neck where much tension was felt. Petrissage using the fingers and thumbs was used all over the scalp area to release the tightness and help with the headaches. Maureen said she felt relaxed and her head felt lighter but her shoulders were very uncomfortable. She has promised to try and give some time to herself over the next week.

Week 2: Maureen commented that she has suffered from a bad headache the next day but that after that she had not had so many. The ache in her shoulders had gone but she still felt very tense and during the massage the therapist found

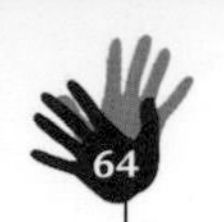

that her arms and neck were extremely tight. The massage therapist concentrated on using kneading movements particularly over the deltoid area and petrissage up the neck. Again petrissage over the scalp area was used to great effect as the therapist felt much tightness.

Week 3: Maureen felt there had been no change from the previous week, still suffering from a bad headache within the first 24 hours of treatment but feeling much better as the week progressed. Maureen had still not resolved any of her family or work worries but she felt much calmer and her shoulders felt much freer. The same massage was performed this week using a much deeper pressure particularly on the deltoid and neck areas to help release any deeper tension.

Week 4: Maureen commented that she had had a much better week this week with only two headaches and these not as intense as they had been previously. A normal on-site massage was given, introducing some hacking and cupping, which Maureen enjoyed as it made her feel invigorated. She felt after the first four weeks that there had been an improvement and that she was better able to cope with life. She was determined to keep up the massage treatments as both a treat and a necessity.

LYMPHATIC DRAINAGE MASSAGE

Client profile

Richard is a 41-year-old bus driver. He is separated from his wife and they have no children. He drinks alcohol every day and tends to eat junk food and snacks rather than a healthy diet because after a long shift he doesn't want to cook. He rarely drinks water or exercises. He has noticed that his face and arms have become puffy and a friend suggested that lymphatic drainage massage might help.

Summary of treatment

Richard had two lymphatic drainage massages. Stationary circles were used to encourage the removal of toxins and effleurage was used to help relax the client. Richard found the movements rather off-putting: he thought the treatment would be more like classic Swedish massage, using harder pressure movements. However, after the first treatment, although he did not follow any of the suggested changes in diet or lifestyle, he felt less heavy and his face was less puffy and red so he was more enthusiastic when he came back for his second treatment. He was reminded that the massage could only clear out toxins temporarily and that if he continued to eat salty, fatty food like crisps and burgers, drink lots of coffee and avoid exercise, the puffiness would return. During the second treatment he seemed more relaxed and able to enjoy the massage. He plans to return for regular lymphatic drainage massage in order to maintain the reduced puffiness.

6 Using massage to treat stress

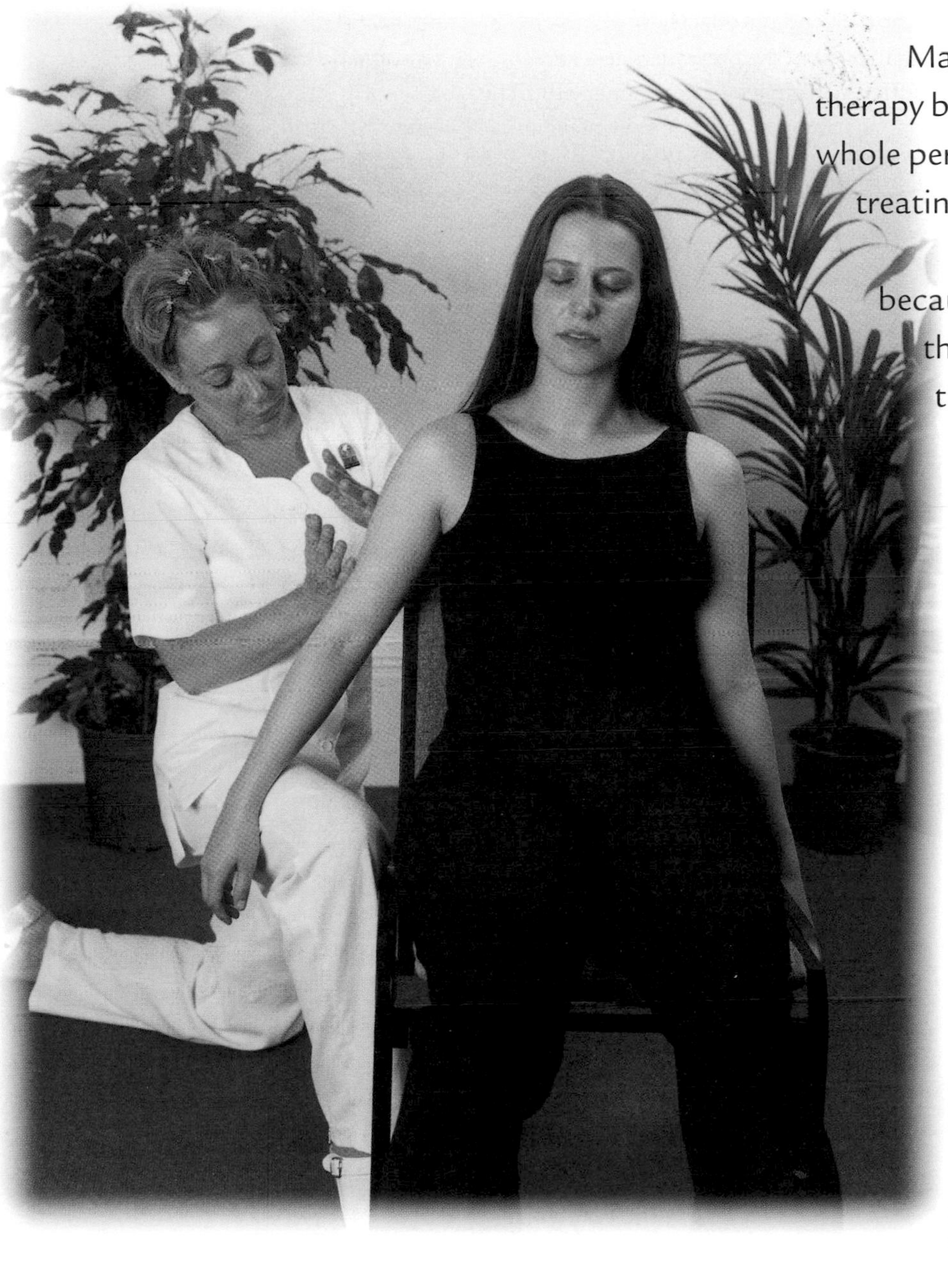

In Brief

Massage is an holistic therapy because it treats the whole person. It is useful for treating stress and stress-related conditions because it helps to relax the body and reduce the effects of stress.

Learning objectives

The target knowledge of this chapter is:
- **definition of the holistic approach**
- **definition of integral biology**
- **definition of stress**
- **how to use massage to treat stress.**

THE HOLISTIC APPROACH & INTEGRAL BIOLOGY

What is the holistic approach?

The term holistic comes from the Greek word 'holos' meaning whole. The holistic approach to treatment takes into account a person's whole being, not just the physical symptoms or problems but also psychology, environment and nutrition and the effects, both positive and negative, that these can have on the body as a whole.

What is integral biology?

Integral biology is the study of our environment's effect on our physical and mental health. Everything we do in our daily lives affects our bodies. For example, an uncomfortable working environment can cause stress, tiredness and related conditions, such as anxiety, depression and heart conditions. At home lack of exercise and a poor diet plus too much sedentary activity (watching TV, writing, reading, using computers) may cause similar problems.

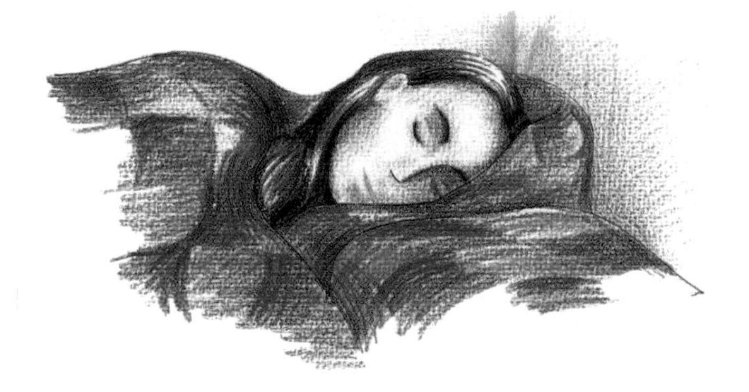

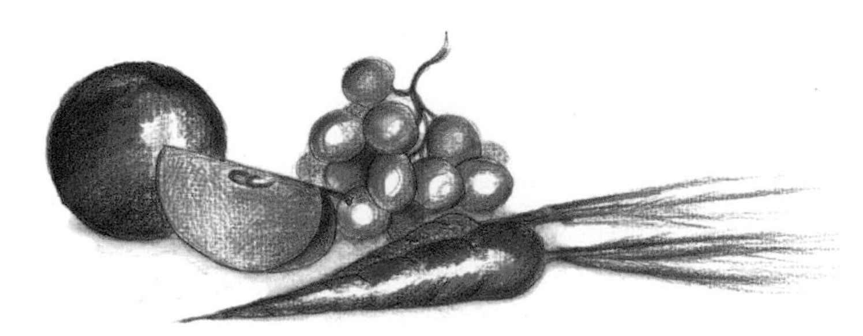

Good health depends on several factors including diet and rest.

What affects integral biology?

There are many factors that influence our integral biology. Some are negative and some positive.

Negative factors

- lack of exercise
- processed food
- chemically-treated fruit and vegetables
- lack of fresh air
- too much alcohol
- a stressful job
- bereavement or grief
- too much caffeine (tea, coffee, cola)
- lack of sleep
- financial problems
- worries about family/relationships
- too much time spent on or near electro-magnetic equipment (computers, photocopiers)
- a smoky or poorly ventilated home or office
- internalising problems and worries.

Positive factors

- regular exercise
- eating fresh (preferably organic or non-chemically treated) fruit and vegetables
- a varied and healthy diet
- drinking lots of water
- taking regular breaks at work and home
- reorganising work patterns to avoid sitting or standing in the same place for several hours in a row
- getting enough sleep
- getting plenty of fresh air and making sure a window is open when someone is smoking.

Why is an holistic approach important?

Because it treats each person individually and in the context of their own life. This enables people to improve their health themselves, thus re-establishing the body's equilibrium, known as homeostasis. For the best therapeutic effect, all aspects of integral biology need to be considered.

You now know about the holistic approach and integral biology. The next section explains stress and how massage can be used to combat it.

STRESS

WHAT IS STRESS?

Stress is any factor that threatens our physical or mental well-being. Such factors can be imagined (worry about the future) or real (financial problems). It is not the factor itself that is damaging but the response to it. Some people have very stressful lives but manage stress so that it does not affect them whereas for others even the slightest worry can have damaging consequences.

There are two types of stress, positive and negative. Positive stress is necessary for some people because it helps them perform to the best of their abilities. For example, most actors and sportspeople will feel, and need, stress before a big performance or event and rather than hinder them, this positive stress helps them to concentrate and focus on the important moment ahead. Negative stress, however, is any factor which causes us to respond by worrying, panicking or losing our concentration.

How does stress affect us?

The body has always had to respond to stress. Thousands of years ago, stress factors were more physical. Humans needed to hunt for their food, protect themselves from wild animals and secure shelter. In the twenty-first century stress factors are likely to be more intangible, e.g. job insecurity, worrying about relationship difficulties or irritation about traffic jams. However, the effects of stress are exactly the same whether the threat is an angry boss or an angry buffalo! The body, perceiving danger, prepares to face it or run away (the fight or flight syndrome). Several systems shut down and the body works to conserve energy to enable movement and escape. Adrenaline rushes into the body to warn of impending danger and the heart rate increases, the blood vessels contract increasing blood pressure, the digestive functions shut down and the muscles contract.

If the perceived danger is then either removed or escaped from, the stress response has achieved its aim and the body relaxes. However, usually, it is not easy to get away from the cause of the stress. Most stress factors are no longer responded to with activity. It is very hard for an office worker to run away from an annoying problem or colleague. As a result the body remains tense and cannot relax. It is this unused response mechanism which is damaging.

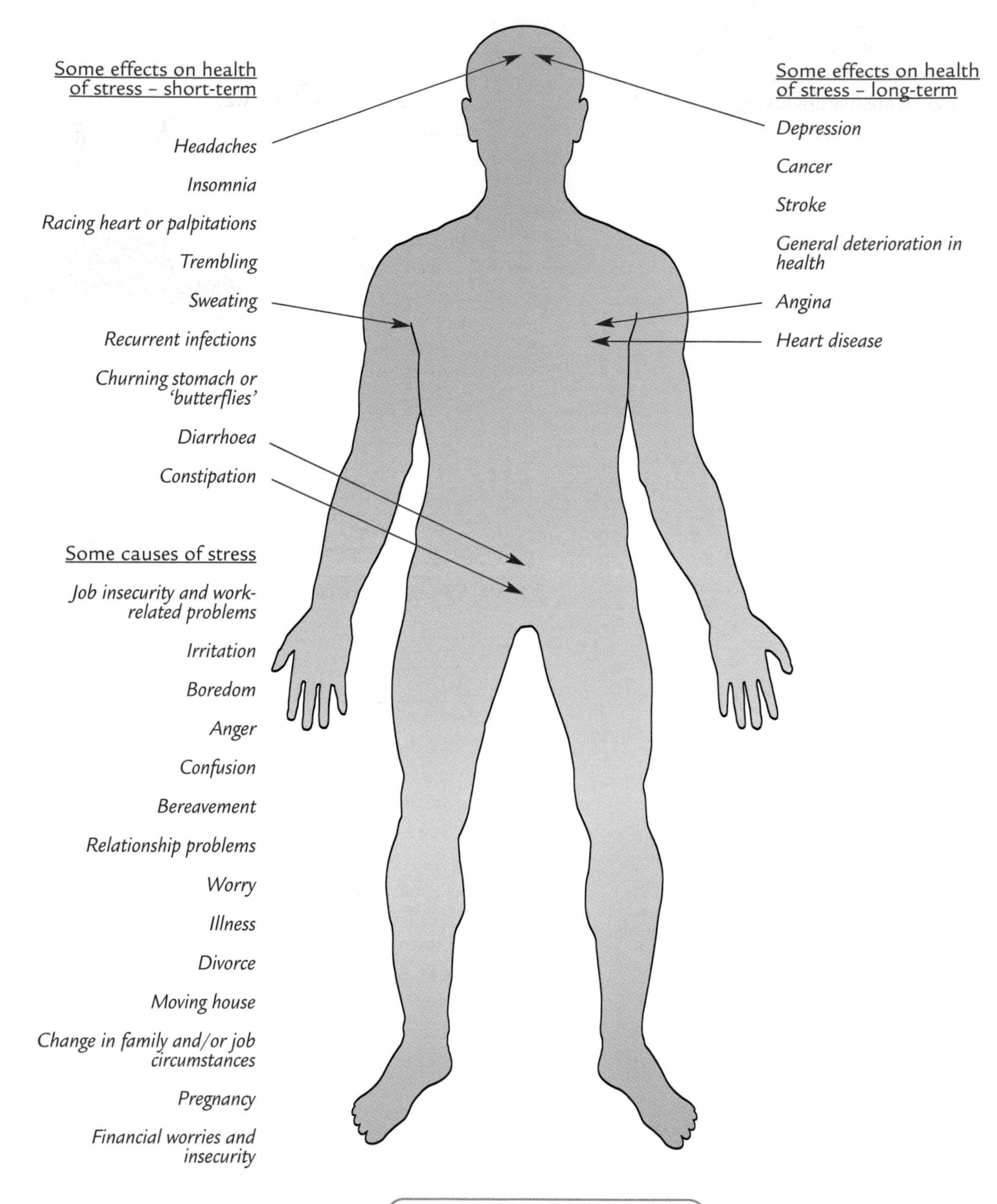

Some causes of stress and their effects

How is stress damaging?

It has been estimated that stress is the cause of 75% of disease. In the short term, as a response to perceived danger, stress is literally life-saving. If we didn't feel stress we would not make the effort to cross the road a little faster to get out of the way of an approaching car, or to perform to the best of our abilities to win a sports match or competition. However, in the long term, if a person continues to feel stress in response to external factors but does nothing either to remove the cause of the stress or to respond to it differently, the stress reaction can be damaging. The body remains in a state of alert and eventually this will have a physical effect on the systems concerned.

What are the symptoms of stress?

Anyone who has ever been nervous about an interview, exam, meeting or important sports event has felt some of the symptoms of stress. These include: churning stomach or 'butterflies', racing heart or palpitations, diarrhoea, loss of appetite, trembling, insomnia, sweating. In the medium term these symptoms, left untreated, may cause chest pains, allergies, persistent insomnia, high blood pressure, abdominal pain, migraines, depression, ulcers, asthma and infections. In the long term constant stress is known to cause heart disease, strokes, cancer and angina.

How can stress be cured?

Stress in itself cannot be 'cured' because threats to our well-being will always exist around us. However, it is not the threat but the way it is perceived and responded to that is most important. If stress is managed, it is no longer damaging, e.g. if stuck in traffic, one driver may become enraged whereas another will accept that this is a normal situation in a busy area. The first driver is responding to stress, the second is managing it. However, the actual stress factor itself is the same.

Meditation

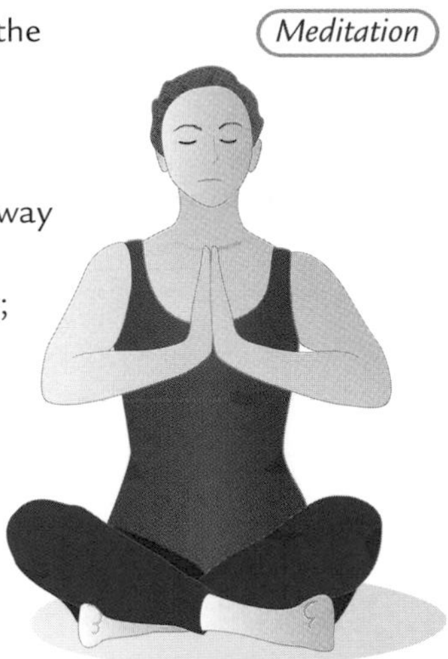

How can stress be managed?

By learning to respond in a healthier way and using relaxation techniques. We cannot simply tell our bodies to relax; we have to learn how to relax them, via relaxing activities, such as walking, seeing friends or going to the cinema, as well as specific breathing, visualisation, relaxation techniques and massage.

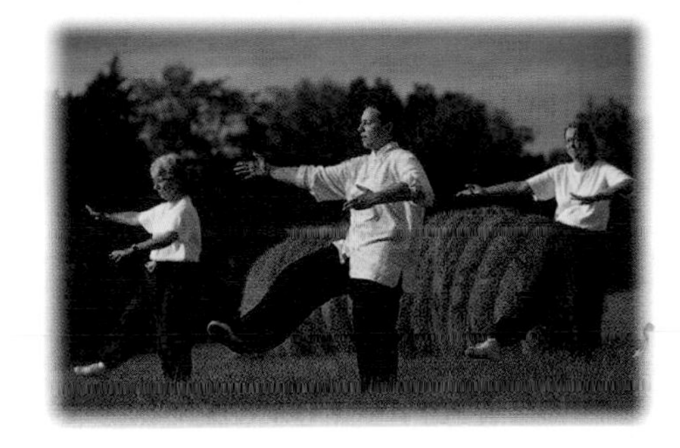

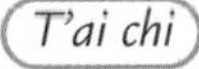

T'ai chi

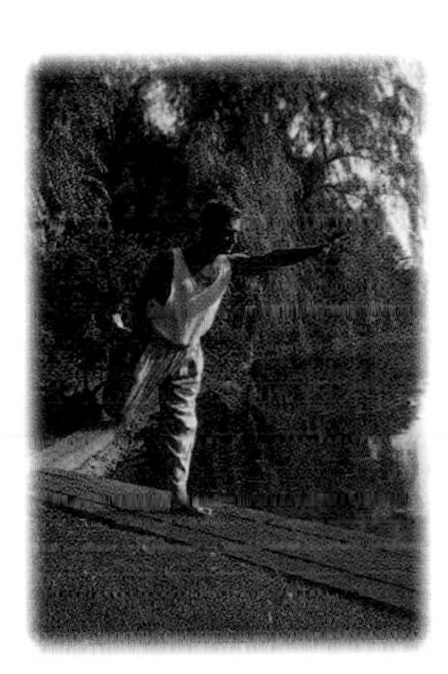

Yoga

How can massage help?

When the body is stressed it must work harder than usual in order to remain balanced. Hence, stressed people tend to over-use conventional relaxation methods such as drinking and smoking in order to be calm. However, too much alcohol or nicotine can have an adverse effect on the body in the long run whereas an holistic treatment such as massage can help induce deep relaxation, helping to remove the pent-up tension of the stress response, without damaging the body. Furthermore, it is easy to forget what deep relaxation feels like and many clients are unaware of how much tension they hold in their body. By relaxing them properly, massage enables them to be more aware of what tension feels like

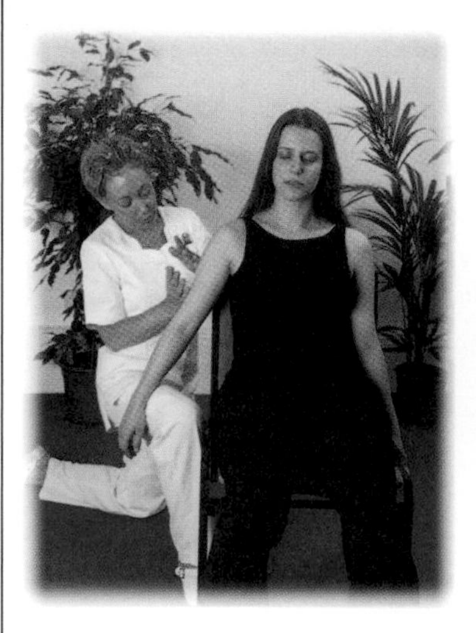

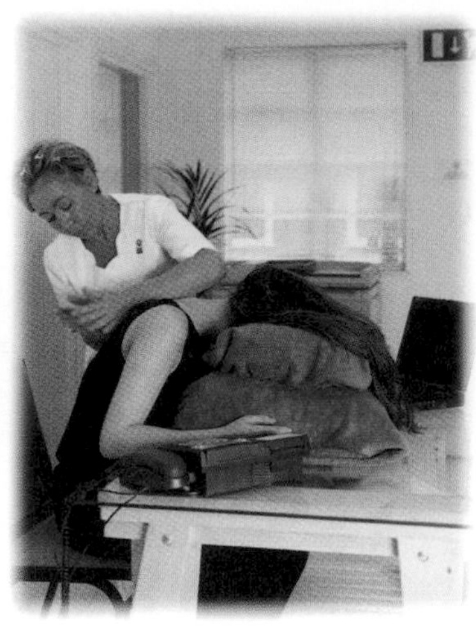

Using massage in the workplace

which in turn helps them to release it. Massage also enables the client to avoid stress altogether. When the body is relaxed problems and events tend to seem less daunting so the client will not feel as threatened and stressed, which in turn will prevent tension building up.

How does massage treat stress and its effects?

Massage treats stress in several ways:

- it is a treatment that relies on touch, one of the most neglected senses. The touch sustained through massage can boost self-esteem and comfort the lonely or bereaved.
- it boosts the immune system, which is weakened by constant stress, stimulates the circulation and the lymphatic system, increases energy levels and induces calm in both mind and body.
- it releases endorphins, the pain-relieving happy hormones.
- it stimulates the parasympathetic nervous system, which slows the body down, encourages deeper breathing, lowers heart rate and switches digestion back on.
- it relaxes all the systems of the body, which either shut down or speed up when stressed, and thus helps with stress-related conditions such as insomnia, headaches, backache and constipation.
- it helps treat depression and symptoms such as low self-esteem by boosting well-being which in turn increases self-worth.
- it stimulates the body's natural ability to repair and renew, at cellular level.

Massage for restoring health

Massage can be very useful as part of rehabilitation treatment after illness. Indeed, it has been used for this purpose for thousands of years, ever since the ancient Chinese used amma or massage for maintaining health. It helps to restore fitness and a sense of well-being. Illness weakens the mind and body but it often causes anxiety and insecurity as well, which themselves lead to stress and stress-related illnesses. Furthermore, long periods spent convalescing in bed can cause poor circulation, constipation, loss of muscle tone, stiff and sore joints and dull, congested skin. On a physiological level massage invigorates the body systems, which may have become sluggish or congested, stimulating poor circulation, boosting immunity, helping the removal of waste from the body, improving skin tone and elasticity and helping muscles recover their flexibility and strength. Psychologically, massage can help the patient to feel less anxious about their health and regain a sense of well-being. All treatments should be approved by a GP, particularly after surgery.

You now know about the holistic approach and integral biology, stress and how massage can be used to combat it and help restore health after illness.

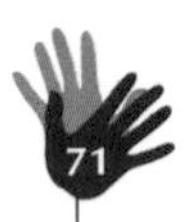

7 Aromatherapy massage

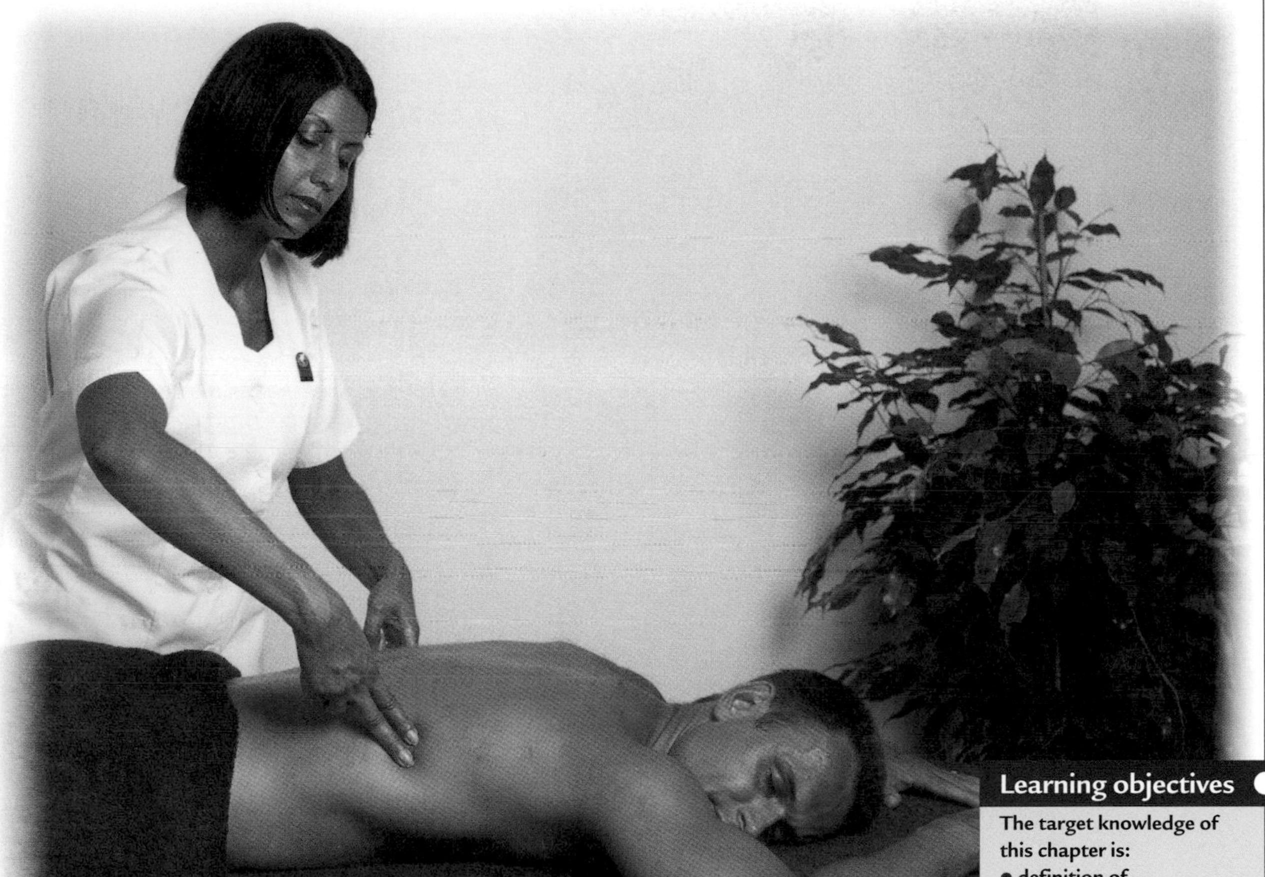

Learning objectives

The target knowledge of this chapter is:
- definition of aromatherapy massage
- how aromatherapy massage works
- definition of an essential oil
- how essential oils affect the body
- definition of a carrier oil
- blending oils
- aromatherapy massage techniques
- when not to use aromatherapy massage
- reactions to treatment and care of the therapist.

In Brief

Aromatherapy massage combines the therapeutic benefits of using essential oils with some Swedish massage techniques.

What is aromatherapy massage?

Aromatherapy massage uses the pharmacological, physical and aromatic effects of essential oils for relaxation and the improvement of physical and emotional well-being. Using a blend of carrier and essential oils in the correct dilutions, the aromatherapist massages an affected area or the whole body depending on the client's requirements.

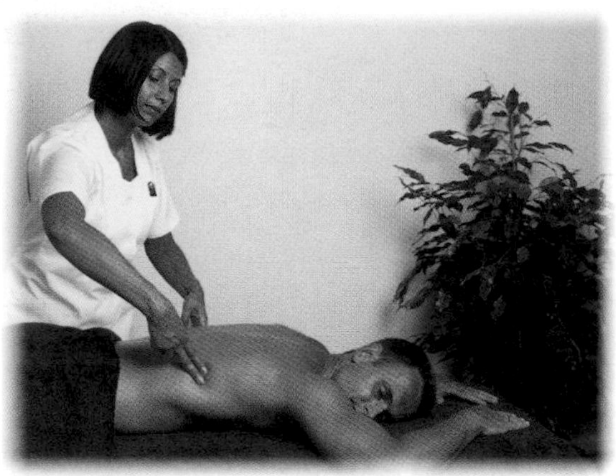

Working pressure points helps release tension

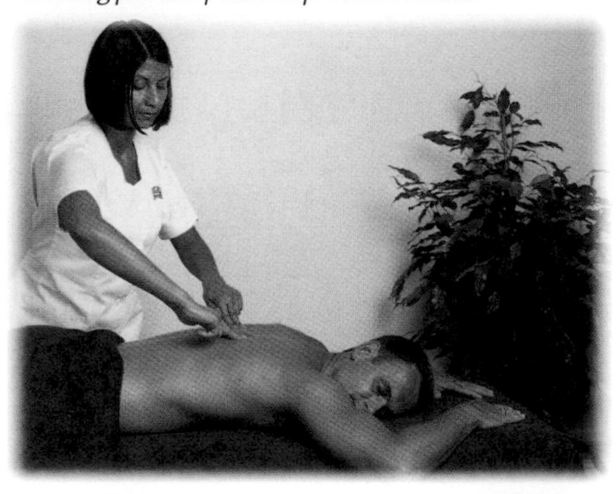

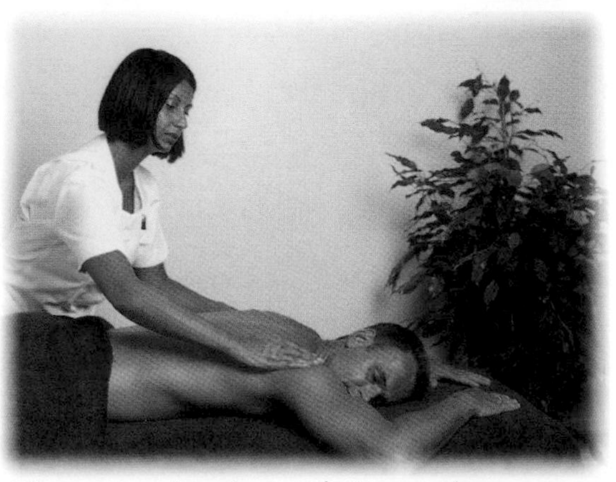

Effleurage is an important stroke in aromatherapy massage

How does aromatherapy massage work?

Aromatherapy massage uses some of the classic Swedish massage techniques to aid relaxation, improve circulation and lymphatic drainage, improve suppleness and aid the release of muscular tension. It combines this with a particular massage medium, a blend of essential oils and carrier oil, to affect the body physically, pharmacologically and psychologically. The warmth of the therapist's hands helps to move the oil across the skin, enabling absorption through the skin and inhalation through the nose. Once the massage oil has been absorbed into the body, the essential oils affect the body in different ways depending on which ones have been used.

What is an essential oil?

An essential oil is an aromatic, volatile substance that is extracted from plant material. It comes from various parts of the plant, such as the flowers, leaves or bark and some plants produce more than one essential oil. These are similar to animal hormones and are sometimes referred to as the plant's life force. Essential oils have tiny molecules and are thus easily absorbed. It is important to use good quality essential oils because their therapeutic benefits derive from their origins and chemical make-up. Adulterated oils (oils that have been changed in some way) and synthetic copies will not have the same effects.

What does it do?

An essential oil has three effects on the body – pharmacological, physiological and psychological.

- **Pharmacological**

Essential oils are chemical substances and so are humans. Once an essential oil is absorbed into the body, its chemicals enter the bloodstream, and are circulated around the rest of the body, where they interact with our own chemistry. For example, the nervous system relies on messages from all over the body, delivered by neurotransmitters along the length of our nerves. These neurotransmitters are chemicals and their messages will be subtly altered by the presence of an essential oil.

- **Physiological**

The way our body works is known as its physiology. Essential oils have an effect on this because they interact with the chemical messages and impulses that our body uses to work. An essential oil with sedative properties will thus send a sedating message around the body, soothing nerves and helping relaxation.

- **Psychological**

As well as being absorbed by the skin the essential oil is inhaled through the nose and into the olfactory tract. The heat of the massage releases the oil's molecules into the air and the nose inhales them. These molecules travel up the nose to the olfactory membranes which connect to the olfactory nerves. Once the molecules have been registered by the membranes and then the nerves, a message travels to the brain. The information is received by the limbic area of the brain, the area associated with memory, emotions and instincts. Smell is thus closely linked to emotions. Depending on the oil and how it is interpreted (e.g. a nice smell, a horrible smell, one associated with a happy holiday) the brain sends different responses around the body. It is thus very important to ensure that the oils used in a massage are chosen in consultation with the client – a massage with a scent that a client dislikes will not be relaxing!

Sweet fennel is a natural diuretic

If they are chemicals, are they safe?

Used properly, essential oils are very safe because they are diluted and only applied in tiny amounts. However, they are extremely concentrated and potentially toxic and should therefore only be used diluted and not applied directly to the skin or taken internally. The following essential oils are not recommended for use under any circumstances:

Aniseed	Arnica
Bitter almond	Bitter fennel
Camphor	Cassia
Cinnamon bark	Dwarf pine
Elecampane	Horseradish
Hyssop	Mustard
Origanum	Pennyroyal
Rue	Sage
Sassafras	Savin
Savory (winter and summer)	
Southernwood	Tansy
Thuja	Wintergreen
Wormseed	Wormwood

You now know what an essential oil is and how it affects the body. The next section explains how to blend oils and the techniques used in aromatherapy massage.

Sweet marjoram is a soothing and comforting oil

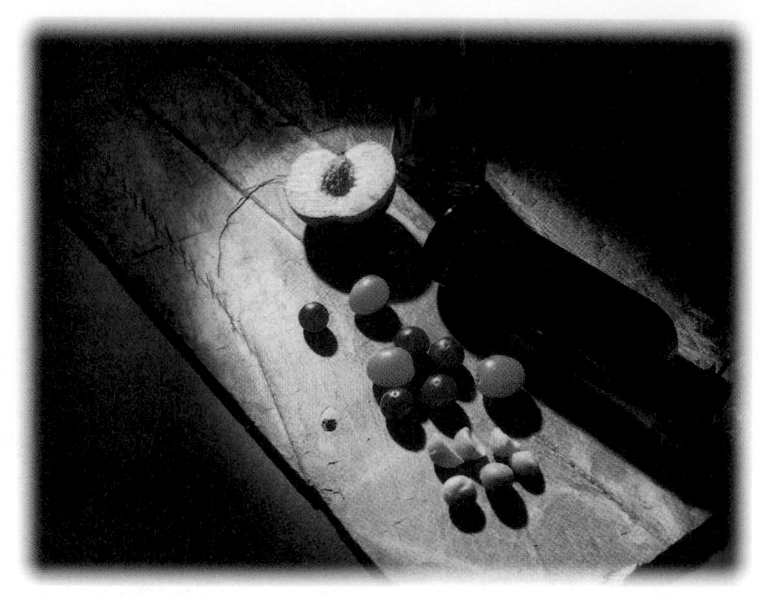

How much of each type of oil should be used in a blend?

The essential oil should be blended with the chosen carrier oil in the following dilutions:

- 2 drops of essential oil to 5ml (1 teaspoon) carrier oil for adults
- 1 drop of essential oil to 5ml (1 teaspoon) carrier oil for the elderly/ frail, babies or children
- 6 drops of essential oil to 15ml (three teaspoons or 1 tablespoon) carrier oil
- 1ml of essential oil to 50ml (10 teaspoons) carrier oil.

No more than eight drops of essential oil should be used per treatment.

What is a carrier oil?

A carrier oil is a base oil which is blended with essential oils to create a massage medium. Carrier oils are usually of plant, vegetable or nut origin and need to be either neutral or without a strong scent so that they do not interfere with the effect of the essential oil. Recommended carrier oils include grapeseed, sweet almond, sunflower and peach kernel. Mineral oils such as baby oil are not recommended for use.

Why use a carrier oil?

Essential oils are concentrated and therefore expensive. It is dangerous to use them undiluted on the skin because they are so strong and potentially toxic. Finally, the word oil in the name is a bit of a misnomer: an essential oil is really the essence of a plant, a non-greasy, volatile substance which would not go very far in a massage. The carrier oil literally carries the essence and spreads it all over the body in a safely diluted and affordable form. The carrier oil has large molecules and is therefore not so easily absorbed by the skin.

Once blended, essential oils will share the shelf life of the carrier oil they are mixed with, but as they are volatile it is best not to mix more than is needed. The following suggested amounts will obviously need to be adapted for smaller/larger frames, children and the elderly:

- a face massage requires 5ml carrier oil (and only 1 drop essential oil)
- a full body massage requires 20-30 ml carrier oil
- a specific area of the body (e.g. hands, feet, arm, neck) may require from 5-15 ml oil.

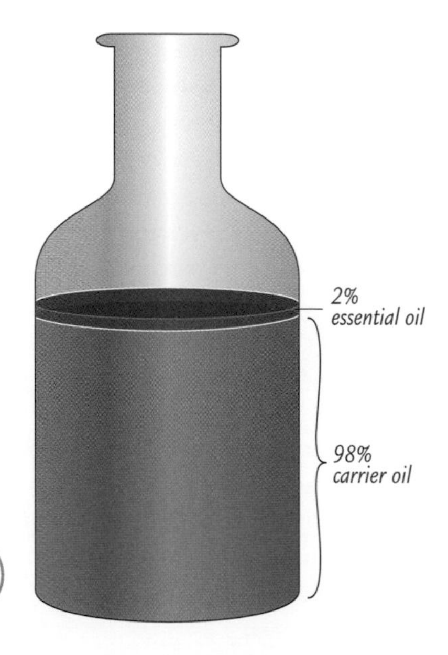

The percentage of essential oil to carrier oil in a normal blend

Which techniques are used in aromatherapy massage?

Since relaxation is the main goal of aromatherapy massage, the main techniques used are effleurage, petrissage, lymph drainage and acupressure.

When is aromatherapy massage not recommended?

As with other massage types there are times when aromatherapy massage is not recommended. The main contra-indications are listed in Chapter 5.

However, with aromatherapy massage particular care should be taken when treating clients who are allergic, atopic, epileptic or pregnant. Pregnancy is contraindicated in the first trimester and from then on mandarin is the only oil recommended for use.

You now know how to use aromatherapy massage and when not to use it. The next section describes the particular practicalities related to aromatherapy massage.

Damask rose is a very effective oil for emotional problems

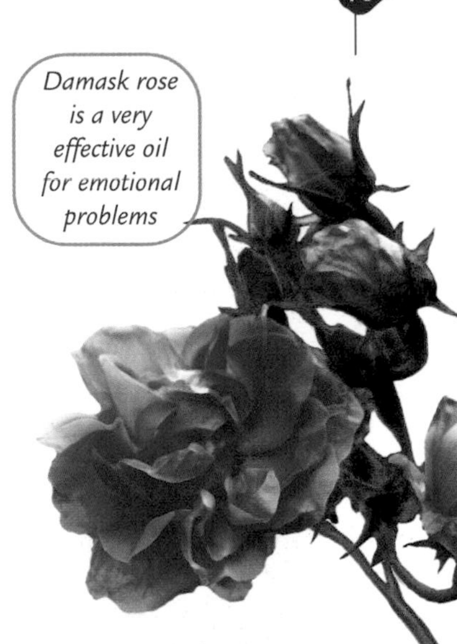

PRACTICALITIES OF AROMATHERAPY MASSAGE

At consultation stage

Discuss the possible essential oils with the client as fully as is necessary (i.e. describing the effects and qualities of the oils, not the chemistry!). The client should smell a couple of oils before you make the final selection. The aroma of the oils, absorbed via the olfactory tract, is vital to the effectiveness of the treatment. Also if there are any selected oils which are unsuitable (due to association or because the client doesn't like the smell) this can be sorted out before the massage begins. It is no good using a blend with geranium on the client if the smell makes him or her feel sick, because the oils will not produce the appropriate therapeutic effect.

Reactions to treatments

When you use essential and carrier oils on the skin you are introducing a foreign substance to the body. In some cases the body may have an adverse or allergic reaction to the oils and this may show on the skin or in other systems of the body (e.g. sneezing or asthma). It is always advisable to be aware that irritations may occur and be able to recognise them.

Non-skin reactions

A client may have any of the following reactions:

- asthma attacks
- migraines
- headaches
- severe nausea
- diarrhoea
- depression
- fatigue
- 'foggy' or 'muzzy' head
- hyperactivity.

Most of these are caused by overdosage. The strength and concentration of essential oils is such that any mistakes in dilutions or blending may cause one or several of the above. If clients are planning to buy their own oils, it is very important to explain that they need to be used diluted not neat (there are very few exceptions). In some cases it may be advisable to provide written instructions on correct use and safety implications.

Preventing reaction

The first precaution is to get as much information from the client as possible and then give them as much information as possible. This should be done in the

WHAT IS LYMPHATIC DRAINAGE MASSAGE?

History

Lymphatic drainage massage was developed by Dr Emil Vodder and his wife Estrid in the 1930s. They worked as masseurs in Cannes in France and many of their clients were English people who had chronic colds and had come to the South of France to escape the damp in England which was considered to be aggravating their condition. Dr Vodder noticed that many of them had swollen lymph glands in their neck and although treatment of the lymphatic system was not recommended at the time due to the lack of knowledge about it, Dr Vodder decided to develop a system for treating it. They later established an institute in Austria.

What is lymphatic drainage massage?

Lymphatic drainage massage is a system of techniques that help the lymphatic system to function effectively.

What does it do?

Lymphatic drainage massage helps to boost the functions of the lymphatic system. It thus improves the circulation of lymph which helps fluid drainage from cells and the elimination of waste, improves the production and distribution of antibodies and lymphocytes (a type of white blood cell) thus boosting immunity from disease and stimulates the lymphatic system's filtering process thus helping remove toxins and bacteria from the body. It also works on the autonomic nervous system, helping to slow the sympathetic nerves (which enable activity) and stimulate the para-sympathetic nerves (which enable relaxation), thus helping relaxation and the reduction of stress.

When should it be used?

To clear congestion, waste and fluid from the system. It is thus indicated for:

- acne
- allergies
- cellulite
- fluid retention
- headaches/migraines
- menopause
- PMS
- respiratory congestion (catarrh)
- stress
- swelling (oedema)
- tiredness

When shouldn't I use lymphatic drainage massage?

Lymphatic drainage massage is contraindicated for:

- arthritis
- asthma
- Bell's Palsy
- cancer
- diabetes
- epilepsy
- heart and circulatory problems
- kidney problems
- lymphoedema
- menstruation
- nerve (inflamed)
- nerve (trapped)
- nervous/psychotic conditions
- osteoporosis
- pregnancy
- rheumatism (acute)
- thyroid problems

Medical permission should be sought before treating a client with any of these conditions.

For more information on contraindications see Chapter 5.

You now know what lymphatic drainage massage is and when to use it. The next section explains how it works and the techniques used.

HOW LYMPHATIC DRAINAGE MASSAGE WORKS

Both types of circulation rely on muscles to act as pumps, particularly in the lower body. All forms of exercise, particularly walking and running help stimulate the circulation by working the muscles and helping the flow of blood and lymph; massage is another form of this stimulation with the added bonus of more focus on areas that need it. When muscles are tired, overworked or damaged they cannot pump as effectively and blood and lymph circulation are therefore not as efficient. This slows down the removal of waste, the distribution of food and oxygen and lowers immunity. At a very simple level this may cause tiredness, swelling and fluid retention. However, in the long term it may cause permanently weakened immunity, congestion of the skin and cells (acne, pimples, cellulite) and lymphoedema.

The techniques of lymphatic drainage massage

Lymphatic drainage massage combines gentle pressure with soft pumping movements in the direction of the lymph nodes. The pressure should never be too heavy because the lymph vessels are superficial and too much pressure is thought to close the valves in the lymph vessels and stop circulation. Softer tissue should be treated with less pressure. All the movements should be carried out slowly. The movements should be performed:

- with zero pressure, thus helping rather than forcing the flow of lymph
- in the direction of the heart and the lymph nodes.

Stationary circles

- Place the fingers of one hand flat on the skin, keeping them close together.
- Without bending the fingers or the wrist, push the skin very lightly around in a circle. The aim is to move the skin not slide across it.
- Always move the skin and apply pressure towards the lymph nodes.

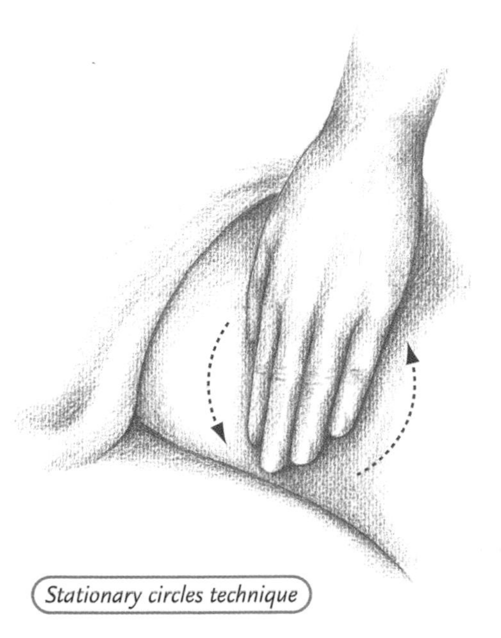
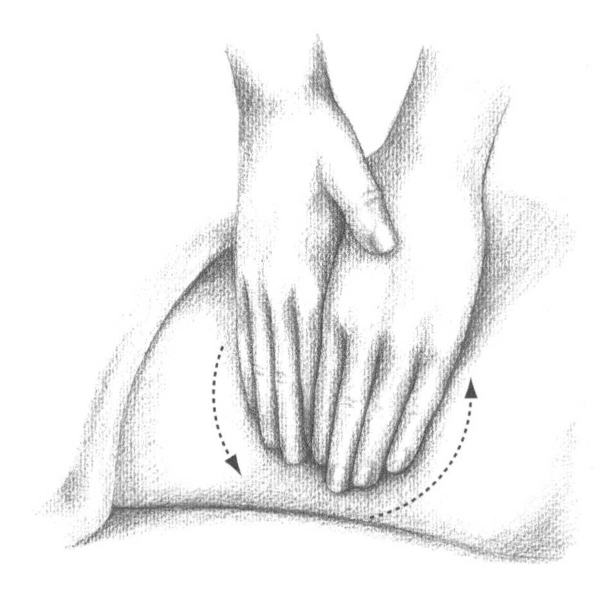

Stationary circles technique

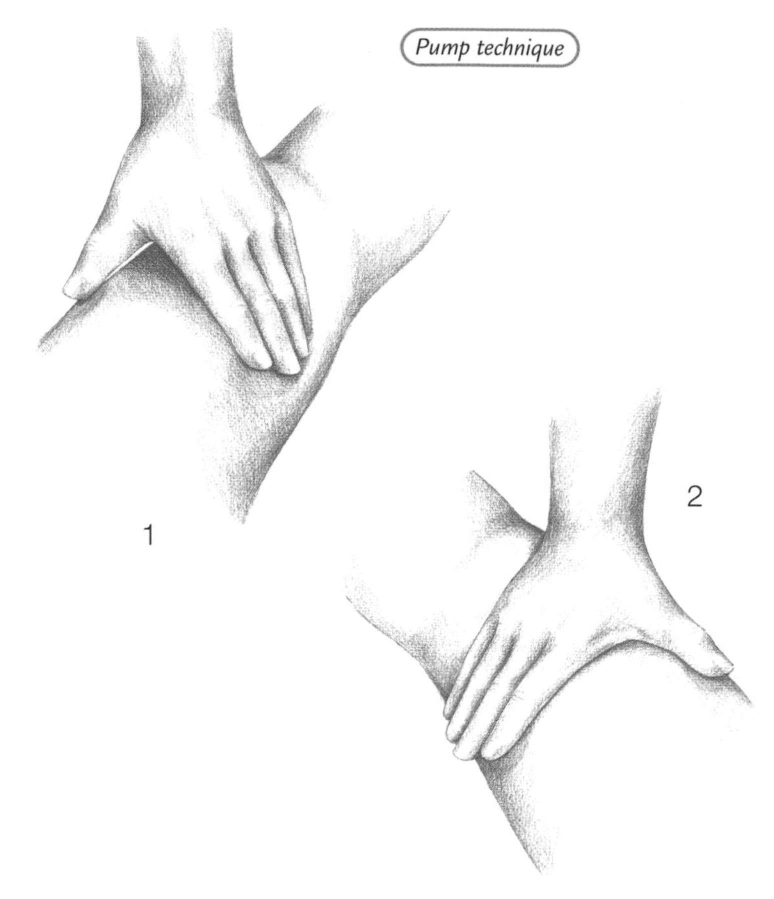

Pump technique

- Place the palm of the hand on the surface of the skin with fingers and thumb separated to form a V-shape and facing in the direction of the lymph nodes, i.e. facing the top of the limb or torso.
- Use the wrist to help move the fingers and pump the tissue. Lift the wrist and palm, keeping the fingers and thumb on the skin (1), and then lower the wrist thus pushing the fingers and thumb forward (2). The V-shape formed by fingers and thumb will gently pump the tissues. Repeat along the length of the limb.
- The movement of the wrist is important. Lifting the wrist away from the skin then dropping it back increases and decreases pressure in the fingers thus causing a pumping movement.
- This technique can be carried out with one hand or both used one after the other.

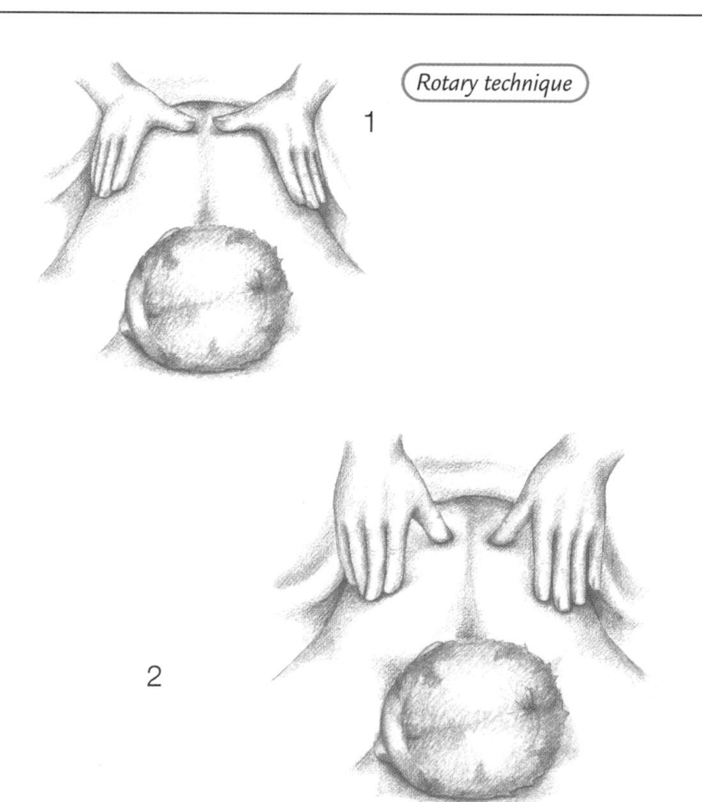

Rotary technique

This technique is used on flatter parts of the body such as the back. Again it relies on the V-shape between the fingers and thumb to push the tissue.

- Place the wrists and hands on the surface of the skin with fingers together but thumbs separated to form a V-shape with fingers (1).
- Push the V-shape of fingers and thumb along the skin.
- Lift the wrists to move the palm of the hand up but keep the fingers and thumbs touching the skin (2).
- Twist the wrist and move it forward so that the fingers and thumb move up the body with the thumb acting as a pivot.
- Lower the wrist and start again.

Scoop technique

This technique uses the whole palm of the hand and is especially useful on limbs.

- Place the hand on the skin with fingers close together and thumb separate (1).
- Move the wrist away from the skin but keep fingers touching
- Move the wrist back towards the skin pushing the fingers up and along the skin with the V-shape join of thumb and fingers acting as a 'scoop' along the skin (2).
- Repeat.
- Move the wrist towards the body to apply pressure and away from the body to reduce pressure.

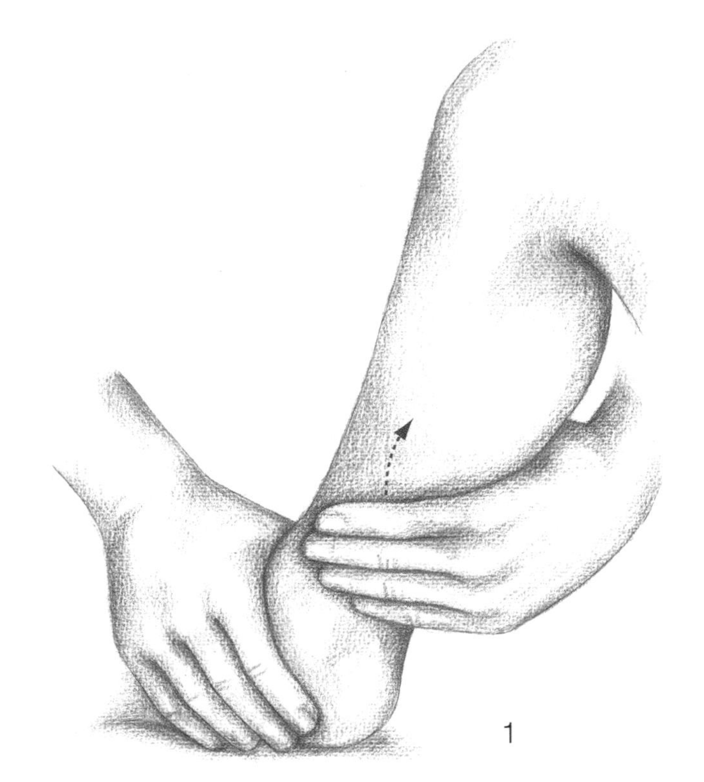

1

Scoop technique: start at the bottom of the limb...

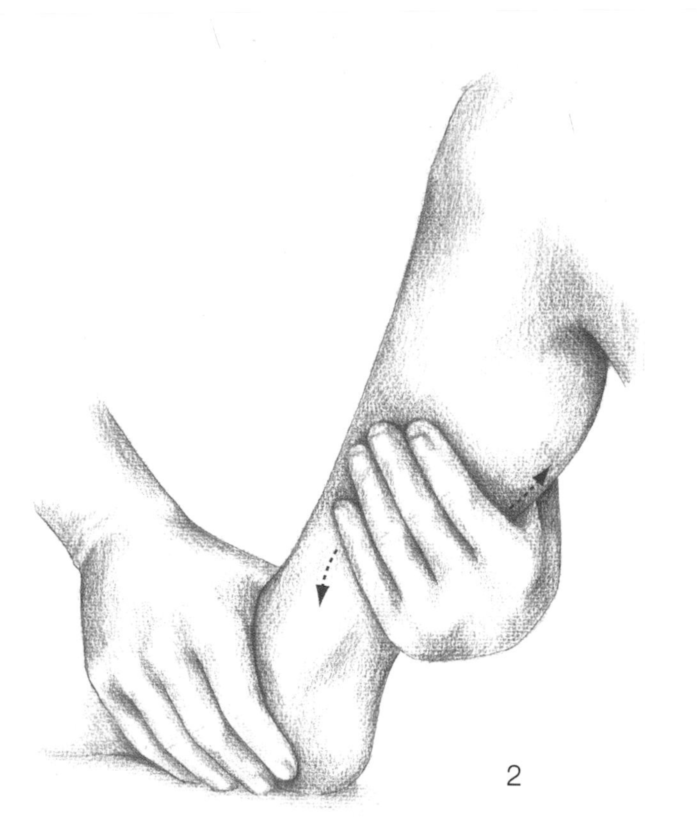

2

... and move up

Thumb circles

This technique is similar to the friction rub used in Swedish massage in that it is very focused and is useful for work on smaller areas.

- Place thumb on skin with tip facing up the limb in the direction of the heart and lymph nodes.
- Turn thumb to the left/right depending on the hand worked so that it is now facing horizontally across the limb.
- Move the thumb back up to its original position pushing the skin lightly along and up.
- The thumb should push the skin not slide across it so the skin should not be slippery or oily. Use a little talc if a drier surface is required.
- Make sure that the skin always moves up and is not dragged back or down.
- Use one thumb at a time or both alternately.

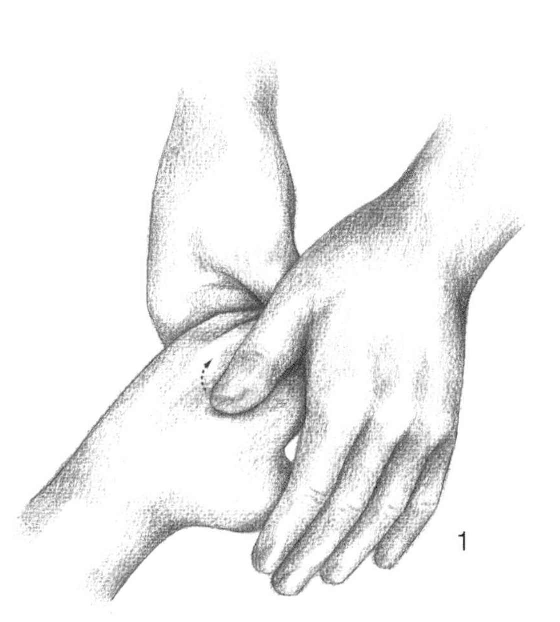

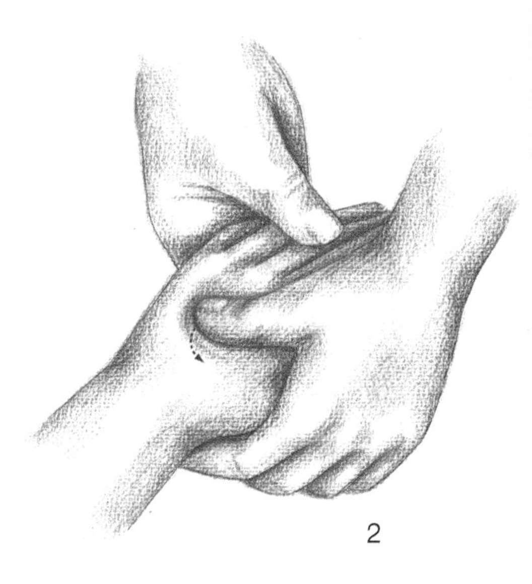

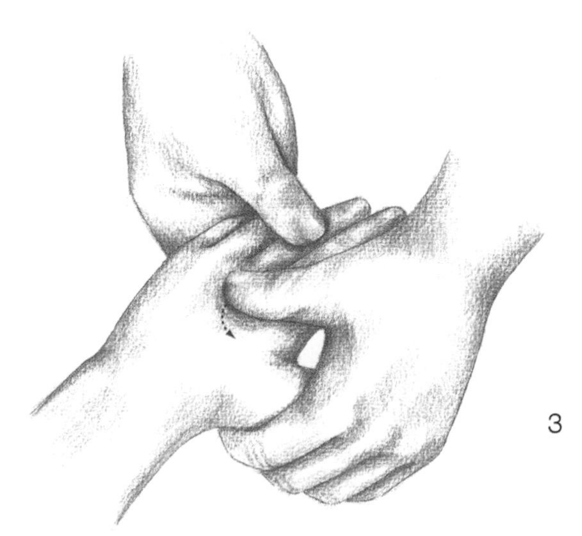

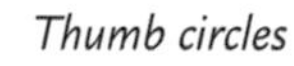
Thumb circles

You now know the different techniques used in lymphatic drainage massage. The next section explains how it affects different systems of the body.

What are the effects of lymphatic drainage massage?

The lymphatic system is a secondary circulation which helps support the blood by collecting and filtering excess tissue fluid from cells. Like all the systems in the body, it has an effect on the others. Therefore, treating it with massage will not only help it function properly but also improve the function of other body systems.

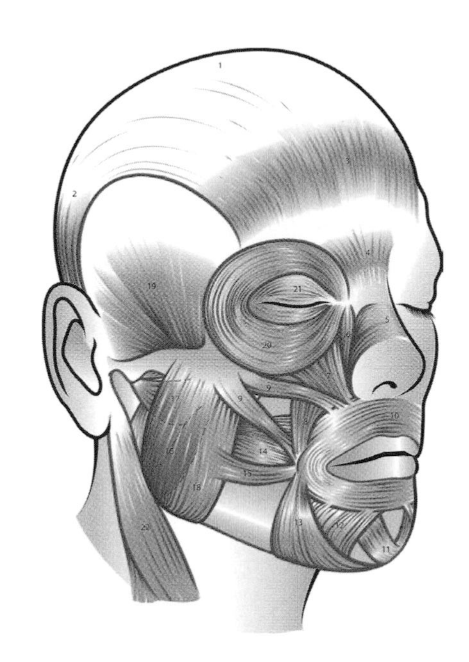

The skin

Skin problems are often caused by inefficient waste removal and the build-up of bacteria. Lymphatic drainage can help eliminate waste and thus decongest the skin, improving its tone and texture and reducing puffiness. The action of massage also encourages desquamation which helps remove dead skin cells, cell regeneration which aids healing and excretion which helps clear toxins from the skin preventing congestion.

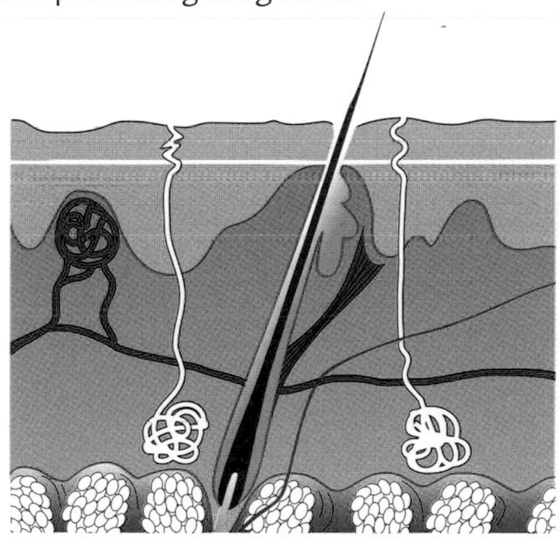

Cross-section of the skin

The muscular system

Waste, particularly lactic acid, prevents muscles from working properly, thus causing them to feel tired, stiff, sore and achy. Lymphatic drainage massage helps speed up the elimination of waste from muscles thus getting rid of the pain and soreness and enabling them to function properly.

The circulatory system

Lymphatic drainage massage helps the lymphatic system to work properly which in turn helps the circulation by removing excess fluid from cells. It is especially important for the removal of excess protein molecules. These are too large to pass through the walls of the venous capillaries and because they retain water they cause fluid retention and bloating. Massaging and promoting lymphatic drainage helps the lymphatic system to collect this excess protein thus helping the circulation to collect any excess water.

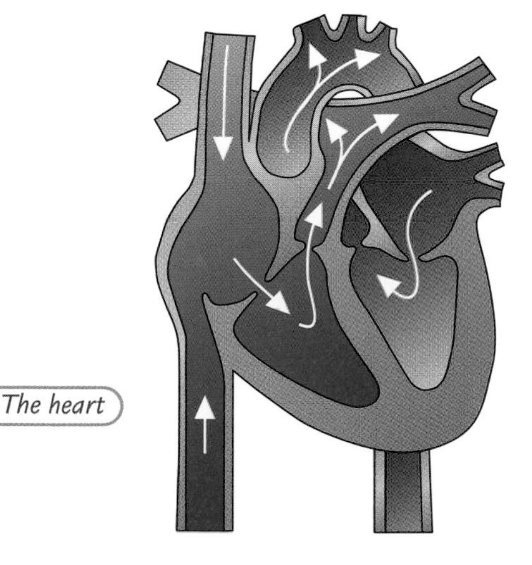

The heart

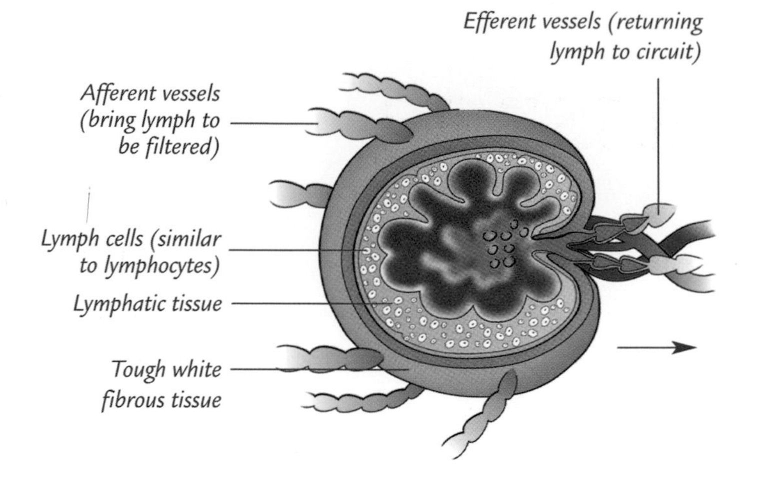

Cross-section of a lymphatic node

The lymphatic system

Lymphatic drainage massage can reduce fluid retention, swelling, puffiness and cellulite which all result from poor lymphatic circulation.

The nervous system

All massage reduces stress and its effects. Poor lymphatic drainage can aggravate stress because it causes the body to feel tired, sluggish and bloated, therefore a lot more energy is required to carry out normal body functions. Stimulating the lymphatic system and helping the body to get back to homeostasis relieves this tiredness and bloating and thus invigorates and energises the client.

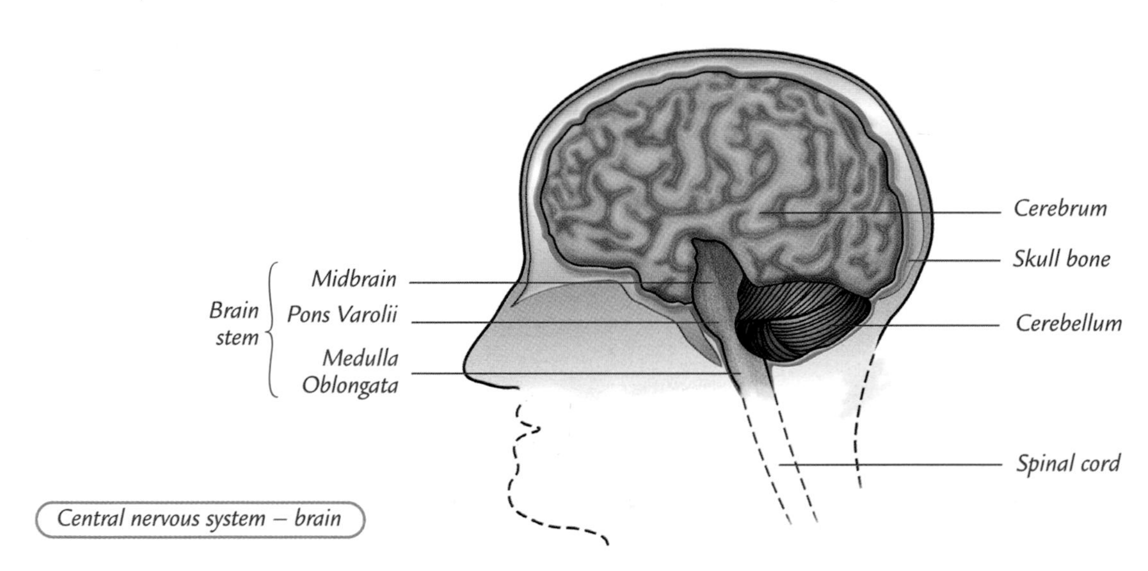

Central nervous system – brain

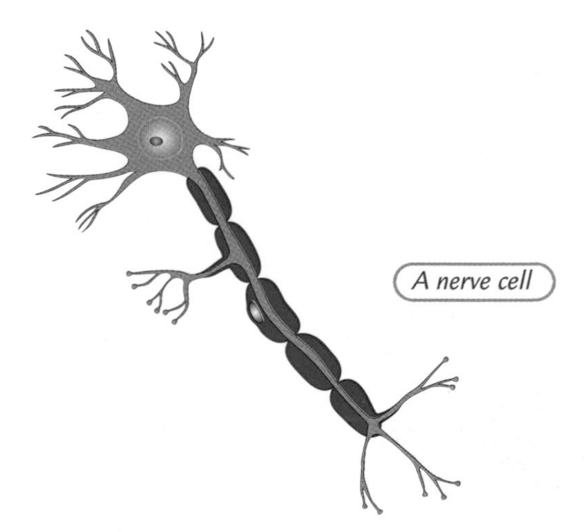

A nerve cell

The immune system

Lymphatic drainage massage stimulates the flow of lymph which, in turn, stimulates the activity of lymphatic tissue, including the production of antibodies. It therefore boosts immunity and helps protect the body against infection.

You now know what lymphatic drainage massage is and how it affects different systems of the body.

9 Sports massage

In Brief

Sports massage combines the use of Swedish massage with additional more intensive techniques, for the prevention and treatment of sports injuries. The first part of this chapter explains what sports massage is, the second explains how to apply it.*

** NB Sports massage therapy is a complex and wide-ranging subject. Within the remit of an introductory guide to massage it is not possible to cover all aspects of this therapy. This chapter therefore offers an introduction to the practical uses and benefits of sports massage, and not a detailed theoretical approach.*

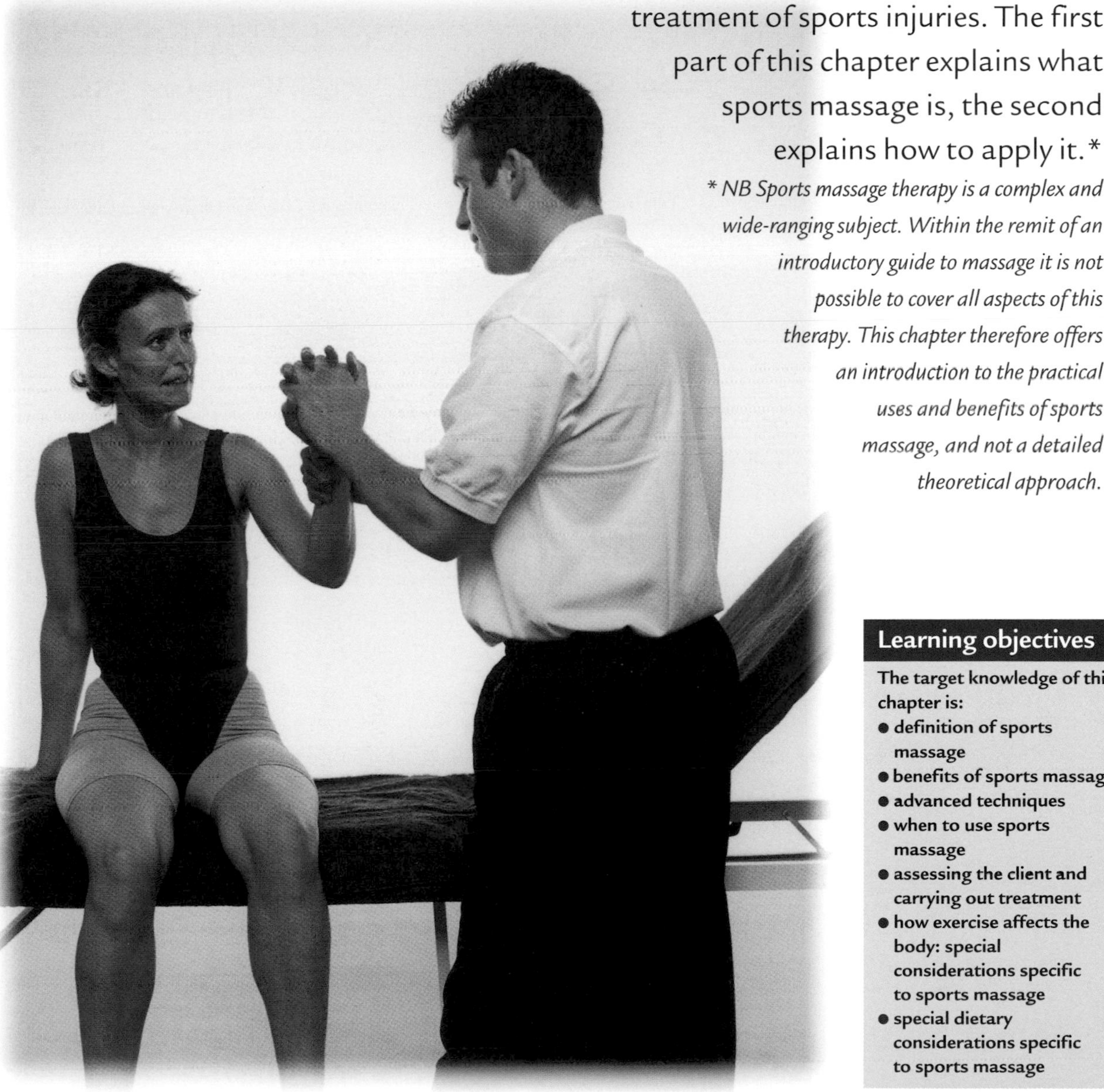

Learning objectives

The target knowledge of this chapter is:

- **definition of sports massage**
- **benefits of sports massage**
- **advanced techniques**
- **when to use sports massage**
- **assessing the client and carrying out treatment**
- **how exercise affects the body: special considerations specific to sports massage**
- **special dietary considerations specific to sports massage**

WHAT IS SPORTS MASSAGE?

Sports massage is the use of massage for the treatment and prevention of sports injuries. It can be used as part of a training programme to help prevent injury, as part of a rehabilitation programme to treat injury, as part of a warm-up for an event and as part of the wind-down after the event.

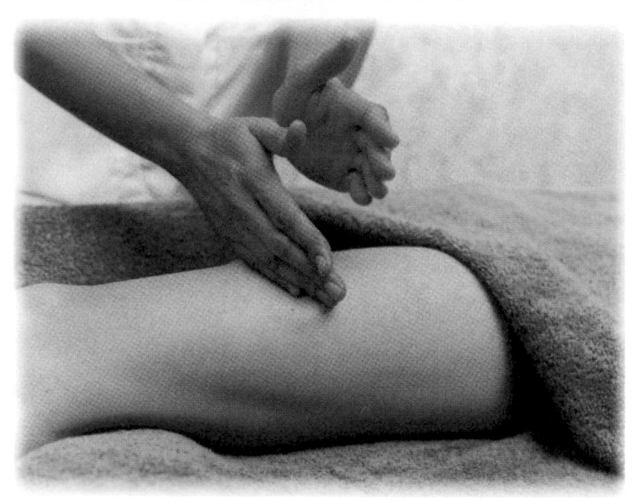

What does it do?

Sports massage, like other forms of massage, helps improve the suppleness and flexibility of muscles and joints. It improves lymph and blood circulation and assists body systems in functioning at their optimum level. Sports massage also has more specific effects and benefits:

- speeds up the healing of damaged or overworked tissue and muscles thus reduces recovery time and allows a sports person to regain their health and performance
- increases fitness capabilities and performance potential
- prevents future injury by identifying and treating current muscle weakness, tiredness and problem areas
- post-event massage helps clear out waste and toxins, e.g. lactic acid from muscles, reducing stiffness and enabling a faster recovery than post-event rest
- massage helps break up adhesions that can develop between the fascia of different muscles, thus improving muscle suppleness and mobility
- enables muscles and joints to heal faster after injury
- improves flexibility
- peak performance can be reached faster and, once reached, sustained over longer periods.

ADVANCED TECHNIQUES

Sports massage combines classic Swedish massage movements such as effleurage with other, more advanced techniques such as lymphatic drainage, compression, frictioning, neuro-muscular technique, muscle energy technique, soft tissue release and connective tissue massage.

Effleurage and petrissage

Sports massage effleurage (stroking) is very similar to effleurage used in other forms of massage. However, in addition to traditional effleurage which is performed using the palms, it may involve the use of the lower arm to apply deeper pressure strokes over larger areas. Petrissage in sports massage relies on the elbow, fist or heel of the hand (the lower part of the palm) to apply the classic kneading movements and deeper pressure to the body.

Lymphatic drainage massage

The lymphatic system is a secondary circulation that helps the circulatory system, the function of which is to drain the tissue spaces of the body of excess fluid. It collects toxins and excess fluid from the cells and tissues, filters off bacteria, produces antibodies and returns the filtered fluid and antibodies to the circulatory system. Lymphatic drainage massage can help the action of the lymphatic system, encouraging the removal of toxins and boosting the immune system. It is useful for treating fluid retention or oedema (swelling). Manual lymphatic drainage uses:

- gentle, pumping movements in the direction of the lymph nodes
- light pressure because many lymph vessels are near the surface of the skin and firm or deep pressure is thought to prevent lymph movement.

See Chapter 8 for more information on lymphatic drainage massage.

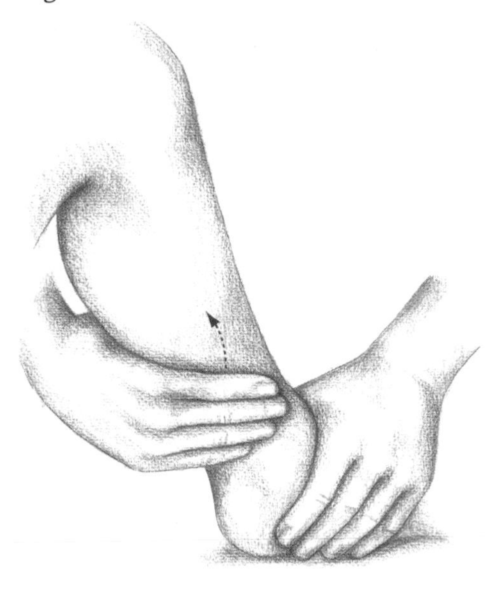

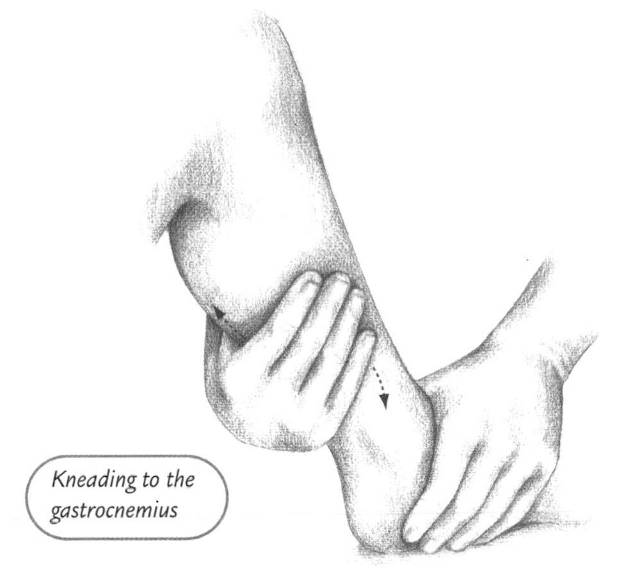

Kneading to the gastrocnemius

Compression

Compression is the application of pressure to the body using the heel of the hand (base of the palm) or the fist to push the muscle tissue against the bone. Like squeezing, compression has a pumping effect, assisting circulation. The therapist should begin pressing at the insertion of the muscle and move along to its origin. It is generally used longitudinally, along the length of a muscle but it can also be used transversally, as with cross-fibre frictions, to help ease stiffness out of a muscle and make it more supple.

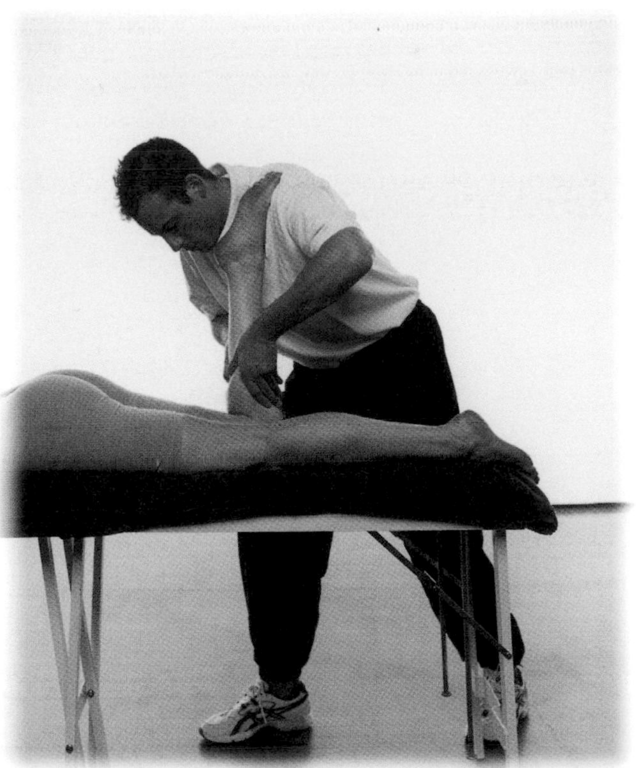

Deep friction also known as cross-fibre friction

Friction in cross-fibre friction is a variant of the friction technique described in Chapter 3. The pads of the thumb(s) and the tips of the fingers or elbows are

placed on the surface of the skin and used to apply firm pressure. The therapist then rubs the skin immediately below the fingers and thumbs, thus moving the surface (subcutaneous) layer of tissue against the deeper layer of tissue. However, whereas friction is usually used along the length of the muscle, cross-fibre works across the muscle (hence the name). This helps to stretch the muscle fibres and release tension. It also allows the therapist to work close to a damaged or inflamed area without touching it because working on one section of muscle helps stretch the rest of the muscle. It is a focused technique generally used to work on a small area. The client may feel discomfort at the start of the friction but the effect should be one of heat and subsequent release, not pain. The therapist may suggest that the client use deep breathing or relaxation techniques to ensure that they do not tense up during the treatment, which would be counterproductive.
Working very closely with the muscles helps to break down any local 'knottiness', lumpiness or adhesions and thus improves muscle function, elasticity and efficiency.

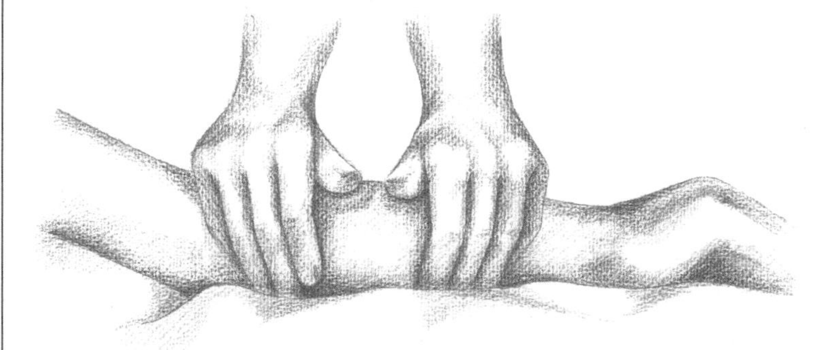

Neuromuscular Technique (NMT)

Neuromuscular technique is a form of friction. However, in this case instead of moving the thumb and/or fingers over an area the digit is held in place over a sore point and pressure is gradually increased up to the limits of the client's pain threshold. It is very important to stress to the client that their feedback is vital so that further damage is not caused. The pressure should be maintained until the pain begins to decrease. In some instances the thumb or finger in use can be circled on the sore area. Deep pressure on a damaged area helps provoke a reflex in the nervous system which helps the muscles relax in the area treated.

Muscle Energy Technique (MET)

Muscle energy technique is a variety of techniques that involve restricted or resistive movement to stretch muscles. These movements require the client to resist the therapist's movements of the joints. The therapist stretches the muscles out until the resistance is felt and before pain and discomfort are felt. Once at that point, the patient should be asked to push gently against the therapist's hold for 5-10 seconds and then released. The therapist will now find further stretching can be achieved without resistance therefore increasing movement. This procedure can be repeated 2-3 times.

Soft Tissue Release (STR)

Soft tissue release combines pressure and movement. Pressure is applied to the area with the muscle relaxed or in shortened position. The muscle is stretched causing the muscle fibres to lengthen and stretch, releasing adhesions or 'stickiness'.

Connective Tissue Massage (CTM)

This is not a massage as such but a form of stretching to release the fluids trapped within the connective tissue between the muscle fibres. Using CTM techniques any

adhesions in the superficial connective tissue layers are broken up and relaxed through reflexes.
No massage medium is used as it only involves stretching using the tips and pads of the fingers, particularly the middle finger. The pressure is dependant upon the angle of the fingers and the depth of the problem area.
For short distances, the middle finger moves along the area taking up the loose skin ensuring a stretching effect is achieved before releasing, allowing the skin to return. For longer distances, more fingers can be used with longer strokes incorporated before releasing.
Pressure can be applied in both directions ensuring rhythm and pressure is constant. Strokes can be repeated between three and ten times to allow for correct skin reaction.
CTM is useful in sports massage when a patient has extremely tender and tight muscles; by releasing the superficial tension the muscle can be softened therefore allowing further massage treatment to proceed.

You now know what sports massage is and the advanced techniques it requires. The next section explains how and when to use it.

USING SPORTS MASSAGE

Which techniques should I use?

The techniques used depend on the client's condition and needs. The five main uses of sports massage – pre-event, post-event, between-event, preventative and corrective – all require a particular treatment.

Pre-event – what is it?

Pre-event massage is used before a sporting event or performance. Its purpose is to stimulate the body (in particular the muscle groups that are most important to the event) and mind of the athlete in order that he or she can perform to their full capacity. It should stimulate the circulation so that all the cells of the body have enough oxygen and nutrients to work at their optimum level and that waste, particularly lactic acid, is rapidly removed and does not build up causing stiffness or cramp. Local circulation will also be stimulated, causing vasodilation and warming the skin and local tissues of the treatment area. Finally, pre-event massage helps prepare the muscular and nervous systems for a co-ordinated response to the athlete's demands. It is part of the warm-up, not a replacement for it.

Which techniques are used?

Providing high stimulation is required, techniques such as petrissage, compression and percussion (hacking and cupping; see Chapter 3), should be used in conjunction with an oil medium. However, relaxation *before* an event may also be necessary to combat nervousness. The therapist should aim for maximum stimulation of the muscles, using brisk, rapid strokes and though petrissage is an integral part of this treatment it should not be used for too long because it may induce relaxation instead of the required invigoration. In addition, the therapist should aim to treat the whole body without working on one area for too long to prevent over-working and fatiguing one section and to keep the athlete warm. The therapist should avoid using relaxing strokes, unless the athlete is tense about the event in which case some slower strokes can be used to lessen the anxiety. Pre-event massage treatment should only be given if the athlete has previously been treated with massage during training or rehabilitation because the massage may disrupt the athlete's performance if he or she is not used to it.

Why use it?

Pre-event massage stimulates the circulation and helps the body to work at its optimum level. Focussing on the specific muscles involved optimises muscle performance and flexibility. It stimulates the mind and body preparing it for the workout ahead.

Post-event massage – what is it?

Post-event massage is used after a sporting event or performance. Treatment should take place as soon as possible after the event, preferably in the first two hours. Most sports, particularly contact sports, will cause some microtrauma to the body, even if only to the skin and superficial tissues. Post-event massage helps to start the healing process required to prevent these microtraumas from becoming problematic. It cleanses the body, ridding it of the waste built up in the muscles during the event and facilitates relaxation and efficient recovery.

Which techniques are used?

Post-event massage should concentrate on compression, effleurage, connective tissue massage and petrissage. These are relaxing and cleansing strokes, helping the body to remove toxins. Superficial and deep effleurage help to push the waste and lactic acid build-up out of the muscles and into the blood and lymph circulation to be removed. Petrissage also helps remove waste as well as focussing on stiff or sore areas, reducing fatigue and soreness and making stiff muscles more supple. Light pressure should be used to prevent further damage to areas overworked or traumatised by exertion and strokes should be soothing and rhythmic both to maintain stimulation to the blood and lymphatic circulation as the athlete cools down as well as to prevent fluid collecting in vessels.

Why use it?

Post-event massage enables a rapid and safe cooling down from the exertion of sport. It may also help to reduce or prevent swelling and help stretch and relax tense muscle fibres. Furthermore, research has proved that post-event massage is three to four times more effective than rest as a way of recovering from muscle fatigue *(see Beck, page 363)*. This is because it stimulates the lymph and blood circulation which helps to remove any lactic acid build-up, thereby reducing muscle fatigue and stiffness. In turn this helps prevent future injury by enabling the muscles to rest properly and heal faster. It can therefore help an athlete to recover from an event and resume their training schedule much more quickly.

Between-event massage – what is it?

This type of massage is used in multiple event situations such as knock-out competitions or pentathlons. It aims to combine both pre-and post-event techniques, thus treating any damage or fatigue as well as preparing the body for the next event.

Why use it?

Between-event massage can speed up the recovery from the preceding event allowing the body to prepare itself more rapidly for the next. It helps to remove any lactic acid build-up, which thus enables efficient muscle function and helps reduce any swelling or complication of any microtrauma suffered.

Preventative massage – what is it?

Preventative massage is the most useful form of sports massage. It forms part of an athlete's training programme and is used to improve general performance and to pinpoint and protect problem areas.

Which techniques are used?

Preventative massage treatment focuses on an overall treatment, combining petrissage, effleurage, percussion, connective tissue massage and friction, as well as more localised treatment for those areas most used by the athlete. For example, a runner would be treated with a general massage with particular focus on the legs using friction and cross-fibre frictions to treat any tight, sore or sticky muscle fibres.

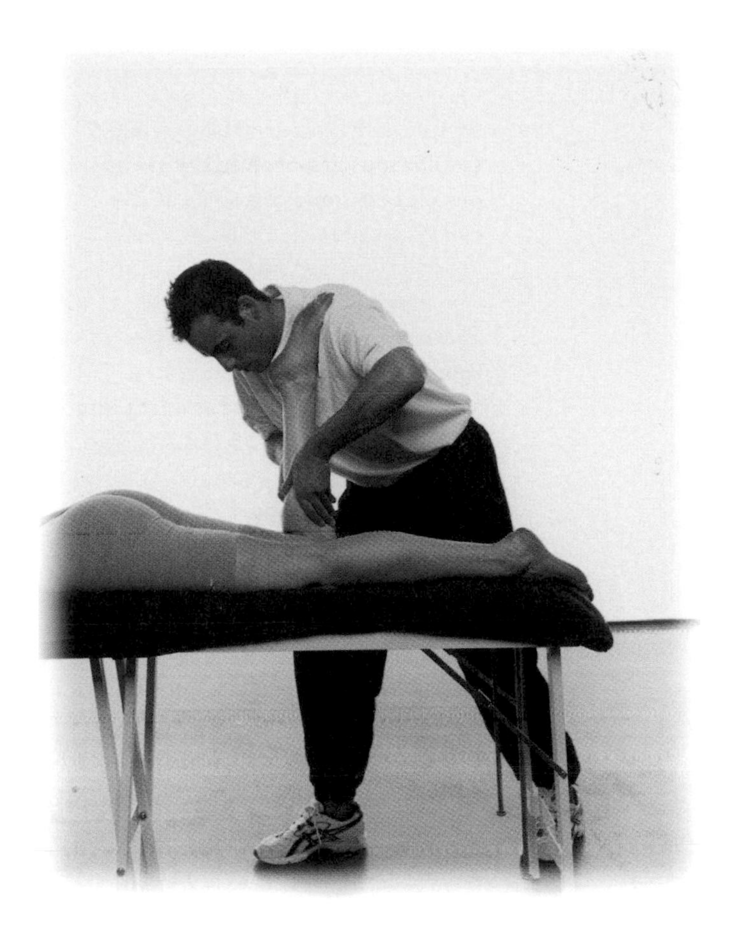

Why use it?

Preventative massage improves blood and lymph circulation, thus improving the delivery of nutrients and oxygen and the removal of waste and carbon dioxide from every cell. This enables muscles to work more efficiently which in turn prevents muscle damage. Massage makes muscles more supple and mobile, reduces stiffness and loosens adhesions thus improving general flexibility and muscle tone, enhancing performance and helping to prevent injury. Finally, preventative massage used as part of training can help identify muscle problems at an early stage, thus reducing the likelihood of performance being affected.

Corrective massage – what is it?

Corrective massage is used as a treatment for injuries. It is the most focused of the four treatments because it pinpoints problem areas, such as past injuries, current injuries or weak spots and those muscle groups most in use and therefore most likely to be damaged.

Which techniques are used?

Frictions, including cross-fibre frictions, compression, petrissage, neuro-muscular technique and vibrations are most useful. Effleurage is more relaxing and should only be used at the beginning and end of treatment, rather than for the more intense work. Pain is an inevitable part of treating damaged tissue but the therapist should not continue to work an area if the discomfort felt is causing the client to tense up. Try applying gentle pressure to a painful area for a few seconds; if the pain doesn't worsen or lessens, then it is generally safe to work the area but otherwise it should be avoided and the client referred to a GP before treatment. This is also a general pre-massage gauge.

Why use it?

Corrective massage enables faster healing of, and recovery from, injuries.

You now know the different techniques and approaches required for the different types of sports massage. The next section explains how to assess the client's needs and carry out treatment.

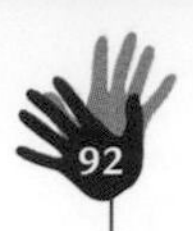

How do I find out where the problems are and what to treat?

For the first massage treatment, the therapist will need to palpate (feel) the client's muscles to look for problem areas, lumpiness, tightness and adhesions. Any pain felt is an indicator of injury or damage to a muscle. Tightness or lumpiness indicates tension or that the muscle has not healed properly after a previous injury. Palpation generally reveals problem areas in superficial muscles; deep muscles are usually inaccessible.

What is palpation?

Palpation is the method used to assess muscles and/or the degree of swelling or damage. Very simply, it is the process of using the palms of the hand (or fingertips for smaller or more tender areas) to touch the different muscles and parts of the body in order to determine their condition. The process is two-way – as the therapist touches the different areas of the body the client needs to explain whether there is any pain or discomfort in the various muscles, so that the therapist can assess the muscle in terms of both how it feels to the touch and how the client feels when it is touched. Generally, the pressure used will depend on the area being assessed – a thigh for example contains many more layers of muscle than a hand and therefore requires more pressure to access the deeper layers. However, sometimes damage is too deep to be felt by the therapist's hands. For assessment of deeper areas, the non-working hand should be used for support because sometimes a reflex action in a muscle other than the one being palpated can suggest a problem. Tension in superficial muscles may also be caused by a problem in a deeper layer of muscle.

Palpation should be carried out slowly, to ensure that the assessment is thorough. The pressure used should be light at the start then gradually increased to prevent any muscle tension developing or causing discomfort to the client. This is especially important on areas that are obviously inflamed or that the client has cited as a problem. Throughout the palpation, the therapist should pay attention to all client feedback, both verbal and physical.

What does a healthy muscle feel like?

Healthy muscles should be smooth, without lumps, spasm or tightness, easy to move and should not hurt when deep effleurage is used. The tendons should be firm but not stiff.

What does a problem area feel like?

Problem areas fall into several categories. When assessing muscles look for the following:

- **tension:** muscle fibres will be difficult to move and not very flexible
- **adhesions:** after injury or inflammation, tissue-making cells, known as fibroblasts, rush to the area and start mending the damage with collagen fibres. In some instances, especially if the muscle remained tense after the injury or healing was not completed properly the new tissue does not receive enough oxygen and nutrients and becomes 'sticky' and inflexible, like scar tissue, and the muscle fibres stick together. In some instances the fibres develop between different muscle fascias sticking them together. As a result the muscles will not be as efficient, other local muscles, bones and joints will adjust and overwork to compensate for the

weakness of the damaged area and the problem, instead of being treated, will become part of the body's structure. Adhesions feel much less smooth than normal tissue.

- **previous injury:** scar tissue is not as mobile or as pliable as normal tissue. Old scar tissue feels lumpy and solid, with little or no flexibility. More recent scar tissue will feel firm with a little flexibility. Wherever damage has occurred the muscles will be rather stiff and inflexible.
- **fatty nodules:** these occur close to the skin's surface and feel lumpy to the touch
- **swelling (oedema):** indicates recent injury or an injury that has not healed properly. The lymph fluid is the body's protection for a damaged area, allowing it to concentrate on sorting out the problem. Swelling can be detected by pressing with a finger on an area that appears swollen then removing the finger: if the finger leaves a white mark in the area oedema is present. Also the affected area will feel watery and full of fluid. Extremely swollen areas will be firmer, even solid, relatively immobile and painful due to the excess fluid pressure on the sensory nerves.
- **painful areas:** try and work out if the pain is caused by any of the above. If not, and if the client themself was unaware of the problem before the massage refer them to a GP before continuing with treatment.
- **inflammation:** look for redness, heat and pain. Superficial inflammation can be treated by working on other areas near the problem. For example, if the inflammation is at one end of a muscle, working the belly and other end will stretch the muscle in the affected area without pain and help it to heal.
- **tear in muscle:** look for a dip or hole in the muscle contour where the fibres are no longer close together. If this occurs, advise client to seek medical attention.

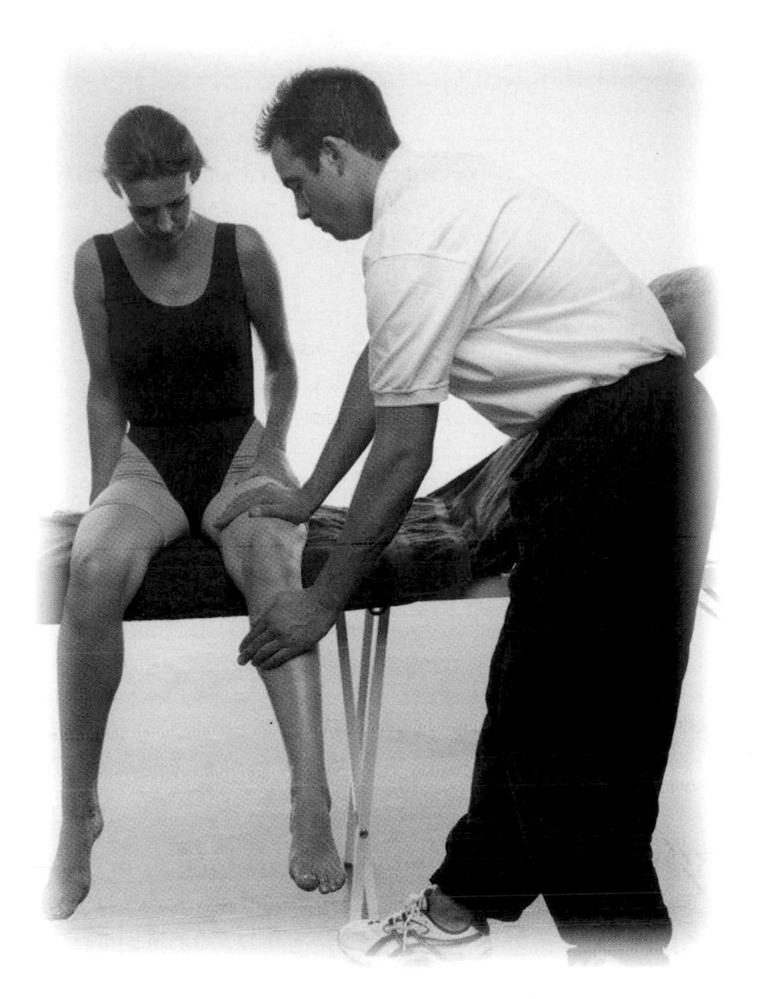

Muscle strength testing

The causes and effects of sports injuries

It is important for therapists to know the causes of sports injuries so that they can tailor the treatment to the actual problem. Consultation and palpation are just as important as treatment because they allow the therapist to find out, both verbally and physically the most likely assessment and thus treatment for a problem. The following table lists the most common sports injuries and their effects.

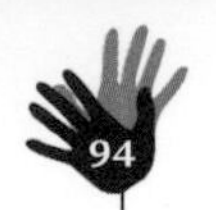

Injury	Cause	Effects
Adhesive capsulitis (frozen shoulder)	Wrenched shoulder, overuse, may follow injury to disc in the neck	Pain and restriction of movement in the shoulder joint.
Calcaneal bursitis	Inflammation of the bursa between the calcaneum and the insertion of the Achilles tendon possibly due to a strain or ill fitting shoes.	Back of the heel feels tender and bruised, no pain when contracting the tendon e.g. standing on or pointing the toes.
Carpal Tunnel Syndrome	Long standing compression found in cycling or from repeated blows in racquet and batting sports.	Acute inflammation of the tendons, causing pressure on the median nerve. Persistent dull ache in thumb and first two fingers, usually worse at night. Lack of grip in the hand.
Chondromalacia patella	Due to repeated minor impacts or occasional major impacts on the knee joint. Also prolonged static or dynamic load on the knee joint during sports like sailing, downhill skiing and weight lifting.	Pain in knee when walking up and down stairs and hills with more pain felt going down
Chronic muscle fatigue	Overuse of muscle fibres which could become irritated and inflamed causing tightness.	Tight muscle causes the athlete to under perform, slows down rate of improvement and could result in injury.
Concussion	Blow to the head – when athlete collides with another and hits his or her head, falls from a height, or sustains a blow on the jaw.	Brief or partial loss of consciousness, breathing may be shallow, face pale, skin cold and clammy, pulse may be rapid and weak, nauseous, lack of memory of what happened.
Cramp	Possible dehydration, lack of glucose, electrolyte imbalance, training faults, fatigue, tight clothing particularly socks and shoes, lactic acid build up and cold weather.	Painful, sustained and involuntary contraction. To help ease the pain apply ice first then slowly stretch the muscle involved apply direct pressure over the muscle trigger point and massage using kneading movements. Contraction of the antagonist muscle will also help to relax the cramped muscle.
Dislocation	Part of the capsule surrounding the joint is torn.	Sudden pain, joint gives way, swelling appears. Sometimes can click back into place, especially in the knee.
Exercise-induced asthma	Exercise makes the respiratory system work faster. For some athletes, exercise may cause exercise-induced asthma i.e. asthma that is specifically provoked by the exercise.	Symptoms are wheezing, difficulty in breathing and/or shortness of breath, a constricted sensation in the chest and, sometimes, coughing. Symptoms usually present about 3–8 minutes after beginning the activity.

Injury	Cause	Effects
Fractures	Can be caused as a result of a direct trauma, e.g. impact on the leg or indirect trauma, e.g. an awkward fall.	Compound fracture – ends of bone pierce the skin. Avulsion fractures – bone attached to a muscle or ligament has been torn away.
Hyperventilation	Abnormal loss of carbon dioxide from the blood, leading to chemical changes within the blood	Unnaturally fast breathing, dizziness, trembling and tingling in the hands
Ilio-tibial band syndrome (Runner's knee)	Prolonged running practice and running on cambered roads	Pain after running a certain distance which increases, causing the runner to stop. Pain disappears after rest but recurs if running is resumed. Often occurs when running downhill.
Jogger's nipple	Clothing constantly rubbing against the nipple whilst running.	Very sore nipple area, in acute cases leading to bleeding of the area.
Lateral epicondylitis	Long standing compression found in cycling or from repeated blows in racquet and batting sports.	Pain is felt over the outer elbow area, increasing in intensity on certain movements that stress the tendon. If severe, pain can be felt all around the elbow, resulting in difficulty in writing.
Mallet finger	Rupture in an extensor tendon on the back of a finger caused by e.g. a ball hitting the finger-tip forcing the finger to flex.	Tenderness felt between the nail and the distal joint in the finger and finger tip held slightly flexed when resting.
Periostitis	Inflammation of the periosteum caused by changing from one playing surface to another.	Pain felt on inside of the bone during activity. As activity intensifies pain increases. There is tenderness and swelling.
Ruptured muscles	Burst or tear in the fascia or sheath surrounding a muscle caused by overstretching, overloading, lack of warm up, or weakness due to previous injury or direct impact.	Swelling, bleeding between the ruptured ends of the muscle fibres, could cause restricted joint mobility if rupture occurs at the joint.
Shin splints or Compartment Syndrome	Training too intensely on a hard surface. Common problem with runners.	Pain mainly down lower two-thirds of shin which increases with continued activity; tibialis anterior muscle may be tender and feel swollen.
Sprain	Stretching and tearing of the ligaments within a joint.	Tissue and ligament damage with local swelling and tenderness.

Injury	Cause	Effects
Stitch	Often caused during exercise or after eating a big meal.	Spasms in the diaphragm; usually occur when the athlete is training or working harder than normal or sometimes if they are under tension due to an important race/game etc.
Strain	Tearing or overstretching of muscle fibres.	Pain and swelling causing restricted use.
Stress fractures	Same as shin splints.	Same as shin splints but if no response to treatment after a few sessions, seek medical advice.
Tendinitis	Overuse of a muscle, causing inflammation and scarring of the tendon	Loss of strength in the muscle.
Torn cartilage	Pressure from the bones of the joint when an abnormal force twists the bones against each other abnormally, causing the cartilage tissue to split.	Instant pain, lack of mobility, swelling, stiffness, and weakness in knee.
Torticollis	Violent turning movements of the neck, eg when diving or when heading or jumping in football.	Severe pain in the neck and between the nape of the neck and the shoulder. Pain on twisting head to one side.

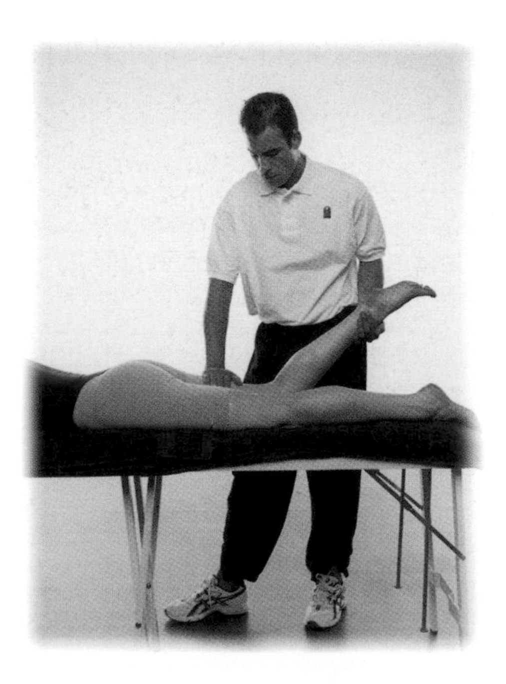

What else should I look for?

Something the client may not be aware of is their posture. At the consultation make sure that you are aware of how they stand and sit. Long-standing postural defects can cause muscle and joint damage. You should also ask about any previous injuries that may have an effect on their body.

Post-treatment procedure

Each individual and each treatment will differ. It would therefore be impossible to suggest a standard post-treatment procedure. However, stretching is always recommended after massage.

HOW EXERCISE AFFECTS THE BODY: SOME SPECIAL CONSIDERATIONS FOR SPORTS MASSAGE

Before treating an athlete or sports person, it helps to understand the effect of exercise and training on different systems of the body. Muscles, for example, need to create energy before that energy can be used in exercise and once the exercise has started by-products from the energy production and muscle use may cause problems such as cramp. Therapists may be treating muscles depleted of energy and overworked. Some muscles will simply be prone to cramp, others will suffer from chronic muscle fatigue. In order to understand how to treat the different muscles worked in exercise it is useful to understand what has happened to them during that exercise session.

How does a muscle move?

Muscles move by contracting. The impulse to contract comes from the nervous system. Motor nerves enter the muscles and split into many nerve endings and each one of these stimulates a single muscle fibre. When the nervous system commands a motor unit (i.e. a motor nerve and all the fibres it supplies) to contract all the muscle fibres of this single motor unit respond together, i.e. 'all-or-nothing'. It is important to remember that the nerve stimulus of one motor unit in the muscle does not mean that the whole muscle is stimulated. For example, at any one time there will be some muscle fibres contracting in all our muscles because this action gives our body normal posture. However, this does not mean that all our muscles are moving – contraction occurs in some muscle fibres even when we think we are still.
In order for contraction to cause movement the contracting muscle needs to be attached to a bone (i.e. it is a skeletal muscle) and pass over a joint. Voluntary muscle (which causes movement and which we control) looks stripey under a microscope. The stripes are made of filaments of proteins called actin and myosin. These proteins run across the muscle fibres in transverse bands. When a muscle contracts the actin filaments slide between the myosin filaments causing a shortening or thickening of the muscle fibres. Fibres shorten when they contract and thus the parts attached to the fibres, such as bones, are pulled in the direction of a contraction and move. Muscles never work in isolation. Any movement is the result of the action of several muscles working together – synergy.
Depending on the number of muscle fibres needed for a particular exercise, e.g. weightlifting, the more muscle fibres are required to lift the weight or carry out the exercise, the more motor units are recruited and in some cases the neural discharge frequency is increased (e.g. if more motor units are involved there will be more 'messages' coming from the brain telling them what to do). When effort is sustained, groups of fibres contract in series.

Where does a muscle get energy from?

In order for contraction to take place in a muscle, there must be an adequate supply of blood to provide oxygen and nutrients and to remove the waste products of energy production. Muscles receive their food and oxygen from the arterial capillaries. This is converted into energy by chemical changes. The main chemical substance produced which provides the energy required is a substance called adenosine

triphosphate (ATP). If the muscle is well-fed and has plenty of oxygen (e.g. a muscle that has not been overworked recently) its cells will be able to produce ATP quickly and efficiently and therefore have plenty of energy. It will be able to work for longer before getting tired. However, if a muscle is lacking nutrients and oxygen it will not be able to produce ATP efficiently, it will therefore lack energy and the muscle cells will not be able to work for very long before getting tired. Thus a sprinter who has just competed is unlikely to have the energy for another run straightaway because their muscles lack oxygen and nutrients and are less efficient at producing ATP and therefore energy.

Muscle cells can store a small amount of ATP but not very much, so it is important for them to continue producing more ATP in order to keep working. Once ATP is depleted the muscle cells replace it using three different chemical reactions – the aerobic system, anaerobic glycolysis and the creatine phosphate system:

- **aerobic system**

When enough oxygen is transported to a muscle cell for its energy needs there is plenty of ATP and thus plenty of energy. For example, when a muscle is resting plenty of oxygen is being delivered to the cell so the cell has plenty of ATP. Most cells contain mitochondria, also known as the 'power houses' of the cell because aerobic energy production (ATP) takes place in the mitochondria. Cells with lots of mitochondria can produce more aerobic energy.

- **anaerobic system**

When there is not enough energy reaching a muscle cell for its energy needs, for example when a muscle is exercising very hard, the muscle relies on anaerobic and creatine phospate systems to provide ATP. Anaerobic energy is still produced in the cell but not in the mitochondria.

- **creatine phosphate**

Creatine phosphate is a molecule that is used to supply energy when both aerobic and anaerobic systems are exhausted. It is a phosphate and when energy is required it creates energy itself so that it can join up with adenosine diphosphate (ADP) (a molecule containing two phosphates) in order to form adenosine triphosphate (ATP) (a molecule containing three phosphates). It can be broken down very quickly in order to help with ATP production.

So how do muscles get energy during exercise?

- **aerobic system**

When exercise begins after rest, muscle cells will use up their small store of ATP for energy production. As the exercise continues and becomes more intense or vigorous (e.g. speeding up on the treadmill or increasing the weight lifted) the heart and lungs try to speed up the delivery of blood, and therefore oxygen and nutrients, to the mitochondria of the muscles in use so that they can produce the required amount of ATP. This is why your breathing rate and pulse increase during exercise – the body is speeding up the functions which increase oxygen intake and delivery.

- **anaerobic system**

The body will, at some stage, (the time when this happens depends on the exercise carried out, the exerciser's fitness level and the genetic make-up of the person) no longer be able to supply the required amount of oxygen to the muscles in use. This is known as the anaerobic or lactic threshold. This threshold is not reached when the body is working to its maximum level (maximum effort) but before this maximum, usually at around 50-85% of possible maximum effort. At this point the muscle must use the anaerobic

system for the production of ATP and energy. The anaerobic system first uses glucose to produce energy. Glucose is a sugar that is stored in the liver in the form of glycogen. When needed it is transported from the liver in the blood to the muscle cells. The muscle then burns the glucose by combining it with oxygen. If the muscles continue to work the anaerobic system will then have to break down creatine phospate in order to produce ATP and thus energy. However, this last stage cannot last for very long because even the muscles of the best-trained athletes can only store enough creatine phospate and ATP for about 10 seconds of exercise at maximal effort.

- **What is maximum effort?**

Maximum effort is measured as follows: it is the amount of weight that one person can lift when all that person's effort goes into that lift i.e. they will not be able to lift it again.

- **Aerobic or anaerobic – which is the most efficient way to produce energy?**

The aerobic system is much more efficient than the anaerobic system. Not only does it produce much more ATP and therefore energy but also its end-products are water and carbon dioxide, neither of which cause muscle fatigue. The by-products of anaerobic ATP production are lactic acid, heat and hydrogen ions. Once the muscle starts to produce lactic acid and other by-products, these products build up in the muscle and prevent the muscle from contracting and functioning properly. However, they cannot be removed until the muscle activity has ceased. Thus, the muscle will soon be unable to contract and the person exercising will feel pain and stiffness. The exerciser will either have to decrease the intensity of the exercise or have a rest.

Finally, when the body is exercising at a rate below the anaerobic (lactic) threshold, i.e. when the body is working at less than 50-85% of maximum effort, ATP is mostly produced by aerobic enzymes which change fat and carbohydrate into energy. However, when the body exercises beyond the anaerobic threshold, ATP is mostly produced by anaerobic enzymes.

How does exercise affect the nervous system?

When the muscles are exercised the nervous system sends impulses to muscles in order to stimulate movement. The hypothalamus in the brain sends a message to the sympathetic nervous system telling it to get the body ready to act. The endocrine system is also stimulated by the hypothalamus to secrete hormones, especially adrenaline. The stimulation of the sympathetic nervous system and the endocrine system has the following effects:

- the cardiovascular system (circulation, respiration and heartbeat) speeds up
- blood is diverted from the skin and internal organs to the muscles so that they have plenty of oxygen for energy production
- the digestive system slows down to prevent wasting energy on food breakdown
- the liver is stimulated to secrete glucose for anaerobic energy production
- the adrenal cortex and medulla are stimulated to secrete hormones, particularly adrenaline which prepares the body for 'fight or flight'
- sweating is stimulated, particularly on the palms of the hands, to help keep the body cool
- salivary glands vasoconstrict (causing a dry mouth feeling)
- pupils of the eyes dilate.

Over-activity of the sympathetic nervous system causes 'nerves' or 'butterflies', a heightened version of the required nervous

stimulation which undermines performance. This problem can be controlled by using deep breathing techniques, using the contraction and relaxation of the diaphragm to slow the action of the different systems. In the first instance, this movement of the abdominal muscles pushes up the diaphragm which in turn pushes up on the lungs and the heart, improving their efficiency. Secondly, the pressure on the heart stimulates the vagus nerve which is attached to it. This nerve is part of the parasympathetic nervous system which slows down the movement and actions of the organs of the body. Thus the heart rate slows down and this has a relaxing effect.

How does exercise affect blood pressure?

The cardiovascular system has to work very hard during exercise. It is therefore no surprise that, though exercise is excellent for the heart and lungs, overdoing it can cause certain cardiovascular problems, such as high or low blood pressure.

Blood pressure

Blood pressure is the force that the blood exerts on the vessel walls as it is pumped from the heart. Without the heart blood would not move. Thus blood is always under pressure. There are two 'types' of blood pressure, which are both used in blood pressure measurements: systolic and diastolic. Systolic is the pressure measured when the heart is contracting, i.e. pressure at its highest whereas diastolic is the pressure measured when the heart is relaxing i.e. pressure at its lowest. Normal systolic blood pressure, measured when a person is resting, is about 120/80 i.e. 120 is systolic pressure and 80 is diastolic.

What happens to blood pressure in sport?

Exercise is known to reduce blood pressure overall and is therefore good for anyone suffering from hypertension. However, care should be taken because during the actual exercise the heart rate increases and thus systolic pressure increases. Sometimes the reading may be above 200. This increase is caused by increased heart rate. Diastolic pressure hardly changes during exercise.

THE IMPORTANCE OF DIET AND FLUIDS

Diet

An athlete's diet (meaning what they eat rather than the control of food intake for weight loss) is extremely important to their performance. Without a balanced diet tailored to their particular physical requirements, their body will not be able to perform at optimum efficiency.

NB This section is a brief introduction, not a comprehensive overview of the dietary considerations for an athlete.

The role of carbohydrates

Carbohydrates are the body's energy providers and therefore the most important food group for exercise. They are preferable to fat and sugar as they release energy slowly (because they take longer to digest) and therefore they can provide energy over a longer period. Carbohydrates are important because they:

- are the most important energy source for working muscles
- help keep the brain and nervous system working properly
- enable the body to use fat more efficiently.

Carbohydrates are stored in the form of glycogen and this store is the body's

most important fuel when exercising. 55-65% of the total calorie intake for any athlete or person exercising should consist of complex carbohydrates such as bread, pasta and cereals which also provide fibre, B vitamins and some trace minerals.
After exercise, carbohydrates are equally important to replace the glycogen that has been used up. Post-exercise is a good time to eat carbohydrates and sugar because the reduced amount of glycogen stimulates the production of glycogen synthase, an enzyme which controls glycogen storage.

What is carbohydrate loading?

Carbohydrate loading is the gradual increase of the amount of carbohydrate consumed in order to increase endurance and therefore performance in certain endurance sports. Over a period of seven days, athletes start eating more and more carbohydrates.This process can boost glycogen stores in muscles by up to 40% - the more glycogen there is in the muscles before exercise, the better the endurance level. Before a competition, usually in the week before an event athletes will start tapering - decreasing their training programmes but increasing their carbohydrate intake.

Which carbohydrates are the best for exercise?

- **Before exercise**: foods which enter the bloodstream slowly and thus provide sustained energy e.g. bananas, pasta, rice (low to moderate glycaemic foods; glycaemic is the rate at which blood glucose rises when a particular carbohydrate food is eaten).
- **During exercise**: energy gels can be eaten because they contain large amounts of sugar which gives instant energy.
- **After exercise**: foods which enter the bloodstream quickly and can therefore be used to replenish energy levels e.g. high glycaemic index foods such as baked potatoes, cornflakes or honey.

Low glycaemic foods, e.g. pulses, apples, green vegetables, etc. may eliminate the need for consuming carbohydrates during long-term exercise because they maintain normal blood sugar levels.

The role of protein

Eating protein is essential to good health. Proteins are the building material for the body and they are converted into amino acids in order to be used wherever required. Protein is found in dairy products, meat, fish and beans. There are some athletes and training regimes which believe that eating more protein than the body needs will improve performance or health because the extra protein becomes muscle. However, there is no benefit to eating more than is necessary – it has not been proven, for example, that protein supplements, which often contain powdered milk and egg or soya protein can increase muscle growth, strength and endurance – and they could even have a negative effect. Once the body has enough protein, any extra is broken down and eliminated. The part of the protein which contains nitrogen is turned into urea in the liver and is then excreted via the urinary system. This may cause dehydration if insufficient fluids are consumed. The rest of the protein is turned into glucose, a sugar, and used as an energy substitute. This energy may be needed immediately or it may be stored as glycogen. But if the athlete already has a full glycogen store, the body will convert any excess glucose into fat.

The role of fats

Fats are made up of glycerol and fatty acids. There are three different groups of fatty acids - saturated, mono-unsaturated and poly-unsaturated. Depending on the way each fat is handled by the body depends on how it affects your health. It is recommended that athletes should eat an intake of 15-30% of fats.

Saturated fatty acids

These are solid and can be found in butter, lard, cheese and meat fat. It is recommended that only 10% of your calorie intake should consist of saturated fatty acids.

Mono-unsaturated fatty acids

These are liquid at room temperature and can solidify in cold temperatures. Examples of these types of fats are found in olive, rapeseed, groundnut, hazelnut and almond oil, avocados, nuts and seeds. These are good fats and can reduce low-density lipoprotein (LDL) cholesterol without affecting the high-density lipoprotein (HDL) cholesterol. It is recommended that an intake of 12% of calorie intake should be mono-unsaturated fats.

Poly-unsaturated fatty acids

These are liquid at both room and cold temperatures and are found in most vegetable oils and oily fish. These fats can reduce LDL cholesterol levels but they can also slightly reduce HDL cholesterol levels, so the recommended calorie intake is 10%.

Some poly-unsaturated fat has to be supplied in our food as they cannot be made in the body. These are called essential fatty acids of which there are two types Omega 3 and Omega 6. Omega 3 fatty acids can be found in vegetable oil e.g. rapeseed, soyabean and linseed oil, oily fish and their oils. Omega 6 fatty acids can be found in vegetable oils e.g. sunflower, safflower and corn oil. These poly-unsaturated fatty acids help in many body functions including blood clotting, inflammation, blood pressure and the immune system. It is recommended that 1-2% of calories in the diet should be essential fatty acids.

FLUID CONSUMPTION

The importance of water

The body is made up of approximately 90% water and is therefore very susceptible to a lack of it.

Water is needed for almost all bodily functions, whether circulation, digestion or excretion. Water:

- forms 90-92% of blood plasma and is therefore essential for blood function – the transport of oxygen and nutrients to cells and the removal of waste such as carbon dioxide and lactic acid
- constitutes 96% of urine and is therefore essential for excretion and removing waste; if urine darkens it means it has a high concentration of waste, which may lead to kidney stones, and this signals a need to drink more water; normal water balance in the body produces pale yellow urine
- enables us to sweat. Sweating is an excretory function which helps control body temperature. When we exercise, muscle heat is absorbed by water, which then dissipates this heat in sweat, thereby regulating body temperature
- is part of saliva and gastric juices and thus helps us digest food
- lubricates joints and protects organs and tissues.

How much water should an athlete drink?

Water should be drunk before, during and after exercise. This prevents dehydration which may cause cramp. An athlete should drink 8 fl ozs/220 ml of water every 15–20 minutes. After exercise, it is important to drink plenty of water to replace the fluid lost through sweating, even if the athlete does not feel thirsty.

What are the symptoms of dehydration?

If you think of how much water the body contains and uses, it is easy to see why a lack of fluid can cause immediate problems. Dehydration can cause chronic fatigue, lethargy and headaches. The cardiovascular system is overworked because the heart has to pump harder in order to transport blood around the body. The volume of blood drops, because there is less fluid available, which means less oxygen can be carried and exercise becomes harder. Finally, because there is less blood the body must choose between sending the blood to the working muscles or sending the blood to the skin to dissipate heat. The transport of blood to the muscles predominates so heat is kept in the body and body temperature increases. It is very important to maintain fluid consumption even without thirst.

Sports drinks

There are two types of sports drinks:

- fluid replacement drinks
- carbohydrate (energy) drinks.

Fluid replacement drinks

These drinks aim to replace lost fluid faster than water. Also, by maintaining blood sugar levels, the extra sugar content helps prevent glycogen stores from being used up. These are dilute solutions of electrolytes (mineral salts dissolved in body fluids, such as chloride and magnesium), particularly sodium and sugars (carbohydrates).

Carbohydrate (energy) drinks

These drinks contain more carbohydrates per 100ml than fluid replacement drinks. The carbohydrate is in the form of maltodextrins (glucose compounds).

What is a hypotonic drink?

A hypotonic drink is a weak solution of sugar and electrolytes and contains fewer particles of sugar and electrolytes than the body's own fluids. It is therefore absorbed faster than water. The amount of sugar in a hypotonic drink is normally less than 4g per 100ml of water. A hypotonic drink helps restore fluids to the body.

What is a hypertonic drink?

A hypertonic drink is the opposite of a hypotonic drink. It is highly concentrated and contains more particles of sugar and electrolytes than the body's own fluids. It is therefore absorbed more slowly than water. The amount of sugar in a hypertonic drink is normally more than 8g per 100ml of water. A hypertonic drink helps restore energy to the body.

What is an isotonic drink?

An isotonic drink has approximately the same number of particles in water as body fluids. The body therefore absorbs it as quickly as, if not quicker than, water. The amount of sugar in an isotonic drink is between 4-8g per 100ml of water which means that it helps to restore both fluid and energy to the body.

Why do some athletes use salt tablets?

Taking salt tablets makes the contents of the stomach extremely hypertonic i.e. concentrated. The stomach will thus absorb any excess fluid in the body in order to dilute the concentration of

sodium. This prevents the stomach from emptying and stops the body from rehydrating. Some athletes think that because they are sweating so much they need to replace the salt but in fact taking these tablets does not have this effect and stops the body getting the fluids it needs.

One way to replace fluids

One way to replace fluids and electrolyte loss is by drinking a dilute sodium/ carbohydrate drink (either hypotonic or isotonic) with a sodium concentration of 40-110 mg/100 ml.

You now know what sports massage is, what special considerations are required in treating sportspeople and some of the problems and injuries that affect athletes.

10 Indian head massage

In Brief

In India massage has been used for thousands of years to treat mind and body. Indian head massage is a combination of ancient techniques and modern awareness of the importance of an holistic approach.

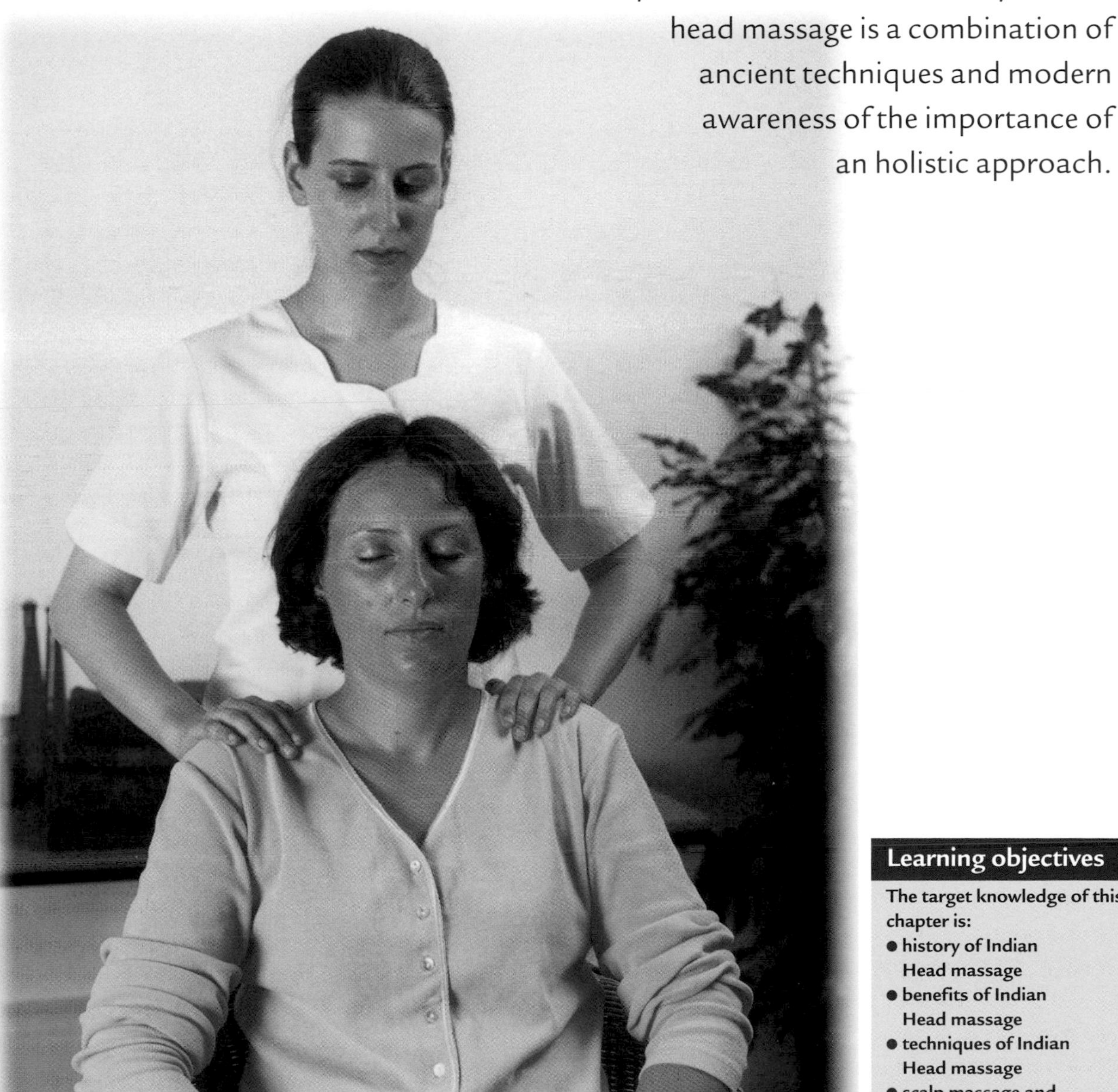

Learning objectives

The target knowledge of this chapter is:

- history of Indian Head massage
- benefits of Indian Head massage
- techniques of Indian Head massage
- scalp massage and using oils
- carrying out a treatment.

THE HISTORY OF INDIAN HEAD MASSAGE

In India Ayurvedic, or traditional, medicine is as important as orthodox medicine. It aims to treat the whole body in order to maintain a balance between the physical, mental and spiritual. Massage has always formed a central part of this. Indian families use massage on a daily basis both for relaxation and healing but also to maintain contact and enjoy the stress-reducing benefits of touch. From an early age children are taught to give head massage so that each family member can both give and receive treatment. At times of ritual, such as weddings and birth, massage has always been important. It is also common for men to receive a head massage when they visit the barber. Over the centuries, practitioners of alternative medicine have recognised the benefits of massage, particularly scalp massage, to relieve tension and stress. In the West the traditional scalp massage used in India has evolved to become Indian Head Massage – a treatment for the scalp, face, neck, shoulders and upper arms.

BENEFITS AND TECHNIQUES

What is Indian head massage?

Indian head massage uses and adapts classic Swedish massage techniques for treating the scalp, face, neck, shoulders and upper arms. It is extremely effective for treating stress because it works on the areas of the body most affected – the shoulders and upper back, neck and head. However, although the treatment focuses on the upper torso and head the effects are felt throughout the mind and body. It is performed on the client whilst clothed, which makes it very effective for short treatments and for treating clients who are uncomfortable about undressing. Oils which have traditionally been used to maintain strong, healthy, shiny hair can be used during the scalp massage but clothing prevents their use during other parts of the treatment.

What does it do?

Indian head massage has the following benefits:

- **skin:** encourages desquamation, and thus improves skin tone and colour.
- **skeletal system:** helps increase joint mobility and flexibility in shoulders, neck and arm. Reduces tension in tissues, making them more flexible which minimises the stress on bones and joints, reducing their need to overwork to compensate for muscles not working properly.
- **muscular system:** improved circulation helps remove waste, particularly lactic acid, from muscles, reducing aches and soreness; petrissage movements on neck and shoulders help reduce tension, stretch the tissues, increase flexibility, release tightness in overworked or tense muscles; stress reduction helps prevent stress-induced muscle spasm in back as well as shoulders and arms; reduction in inflammation or pain.
- **circulatory system:** improves circulation, thus improving the delivery of nutrients and oxygen and speeding up the removal of wastes and toxins; lowers blood pressure.
- **lymphatic system:** improves lymphatic circulation thus speeding up the removal of excess fluid and waste from cells, helping to reduce swelling and reducing the risk of infection through improved production and delivery of white blood cells.

- **nervous system:** reduces effects of stress thus facilitating sleep, reduces anxiety, slows down heart rate, improves breathing, releases physical and mental tension, promotes feelings of calm and well-being; helps unblock congestion throughout the body enabling improved neural communication; release of tension increases energy levels.

How do I do it?

The techniques used in Indian head massage are similar to those used in classic Swedish massage. There are five basic strokes.

Effleurage/Gentle stroking

What is it?

- preparatory and concluding stroke
- gentle and relaxing
- can be used superficially to relax or more deeply, applying more pressure, to stimulate the circulation and energise the client.

What does it do?

- prepares the client's mind and body for the deeper, firmer strokes
- warms the skin
- improves circulation, thereby helping to eliminate toxins from tissues and enabling them to work more efficiently
- relaxes and soothes nerve endings.

Petrissage/Kneading

What is it?

- kneading, squeezing stroke using whole hand or just fingers and thumbs which lifts tissues and muscles away from bones and joints, compresses them and then releases them.

What does it do?

- stretches the muscle fibres and tissues, thereby helping to reduce stiffness, inflexibility and tension
- encourages the elimination of waste and toxins from tissues
- improves circulation
- reduces nervous muscle spasm by helping release tension.

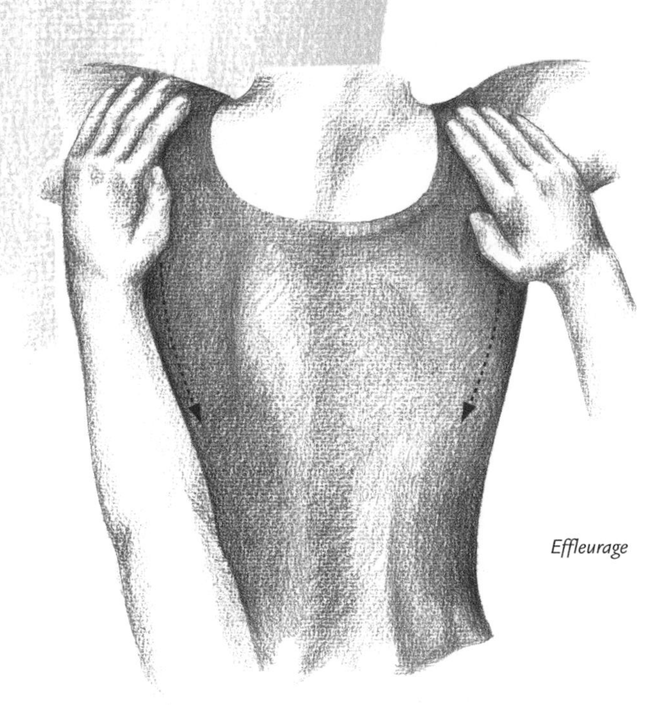

Effleurage

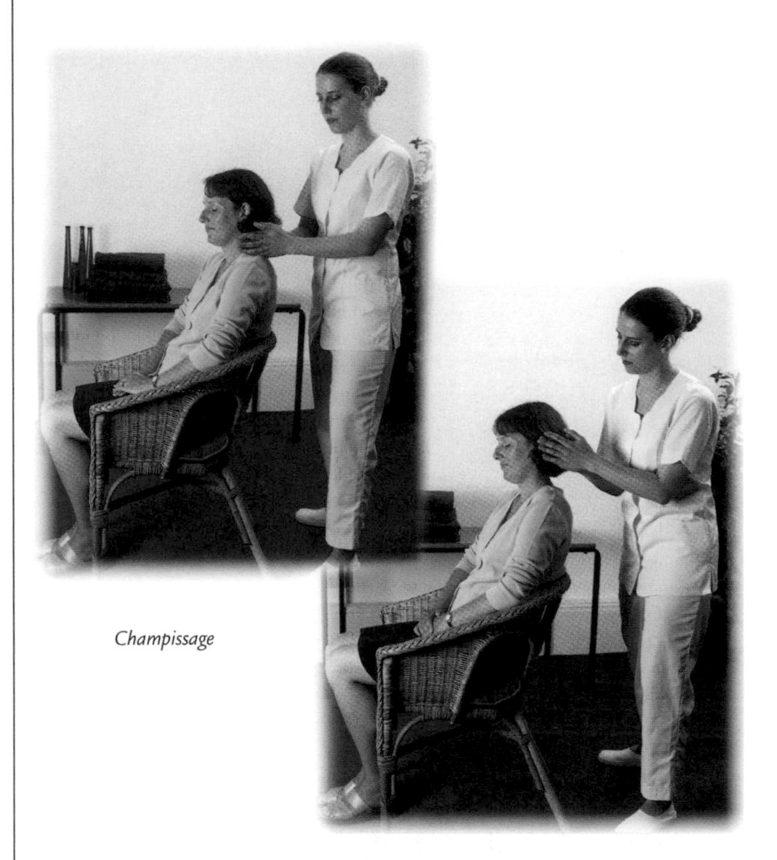

Champissage

Champissage (percussion)

What is it?

- movement using both hands together in a 'prayer' position in a rhythmic hacking movement
- can be used gently to relax or more firmly to energise and 'wake up' the body, particularly the nerves and muscles.

What does it do?

- stimulates the nerves
- improves the circulation
- energises the mind and body and provides a 'wake up'
- improves muscle tone.

Tabla

What is it?

- superficial tapping movement using the tops of the fingers or the heels of the hands
- can be used gently to relax or more firmly to energise and 'wake up' the body, particularly the nerves and muscles.

What does it do?

- stimulates the nerves
- improves the circulation
- energises the mind and body and provides a 'wake up'
- improves muscle tone.

Friction/Rubbing tissue against bone

What is it?

- a rubbing stroke, using either the whole hand or just the fingers, thumbs or palm of the hand, which compresses tissue against bone.

What does it do?

- improves circulation
- improves mobility by releasing tension in muscles
- when used on scalp encourages hair growth
- when used on skin helps desquamation thus improving skin tone and colour and encouraging cell regeneration.
- breaks down scar tissue and stimulates growth of new tissue.

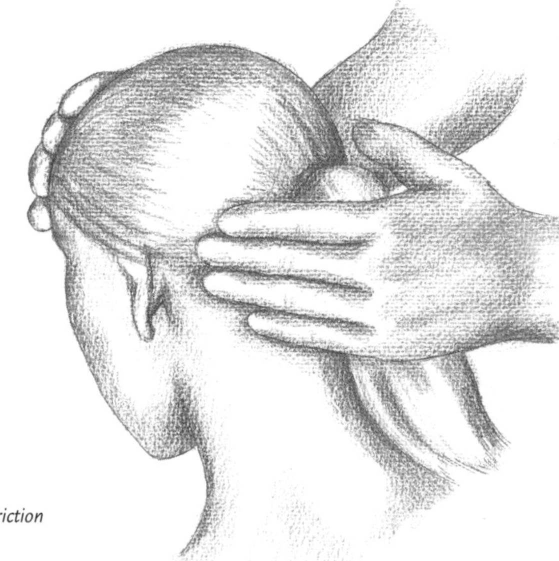

Friction

Pressure points

What is it?

- the application of pressure on specific points using fingertips and thumbs. These points, found along the 'meridians' of the body, release blocked 'energy'. Indian head massage often works on the 'chakras'.

What does it do?

- improves circulation
- encourages decongestion of the whole body thus boosting energy
- stimulates nerves.

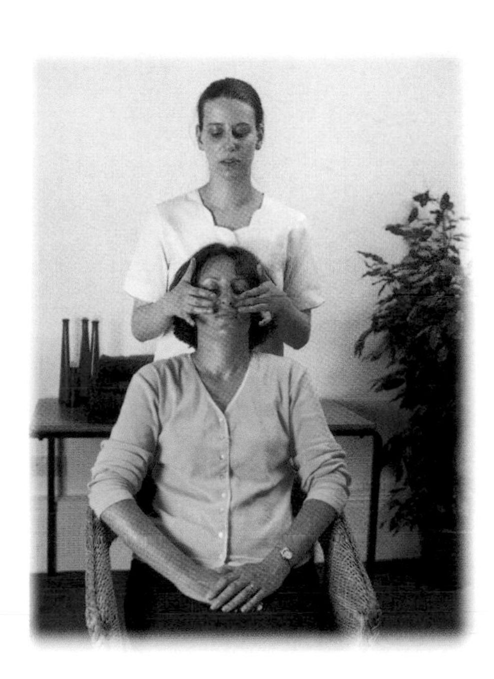

Working pressure points

What is scalp massage

Scalp massage uses specific massage techniques unique to this form of treatment. It stimulates the nerves and the blood supply to the scalp, using a combination of petrissage, friction, pressure and effleurage, and is the only part of Indian head massage where oils are used.

Why use oils?

Using oil conditions the scalp and the hair and adds to the relaxation. Tension sometimes causes hair loss and an oil massage can help stimulate hair growth. Oils are not always necessary or desired and their use will depend on the particular wishes/needs of the client. In some instances essential oils can be blended with a base oil for the scalp massage. The

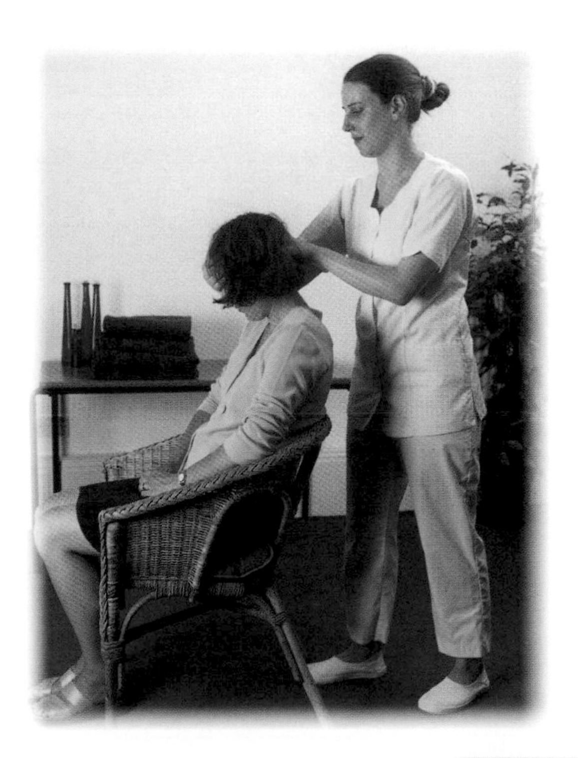

aromatic effects of the oils are enhanced by the fact that they are being used on the head, close to the olfactory tract and thus the oil molecules do not have to travel far. Also the client's breathing will usually be deeper and more relaxed and thus more effective at inhaling the smell.

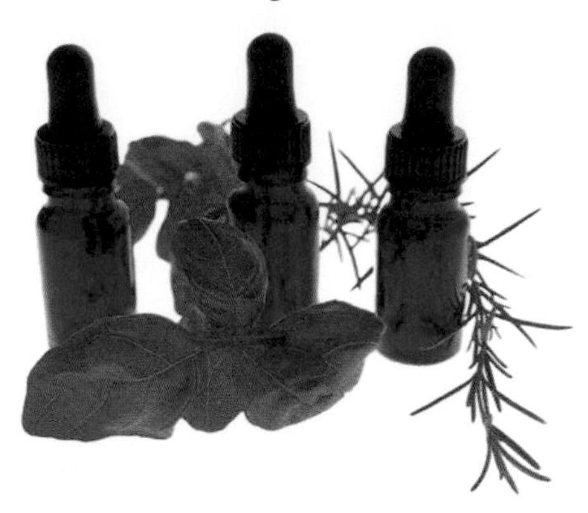

Oils for a basic scalp massage are usually chosen because they moisturise the skin, condition the hair, stimulate hair growth and are neutral in scent. In India mustard oil, almond oil, coconut oil, sesame oil, and olive oil are traditionally used.

Mustard oil

Extracted from Yellow Mustard seeds. This oil is mainly used in north-west India. Mustard oil generates heat, making it popular for use in the cold winter months. It is particularly popular with males. Benefits include:

- stimulates circulation
- reduces pain and swelling
- soothes sore, tense muscles

Almond oil

A popular and easily obtainable oil in the West. Benefits include:

- good for mature skin and dry hair
- reduces muscular aches and pains
- calms the nerves

Coconut oil

Traditionally used by women as it has a sweet odour. Benefits include:

- lubricates dry skin and hair

Sesame oil

The most widely used oil in India. Benefits include:

- moisturises skin and hair
- reduces muscular aches and pains
- reduces swelling
- reduces stiffness
- reduces premature ageing

Olive oil

Benefits include:

- relieves the pain of arthritis
- relieves sore, tense muscles
- reduces swelling

However, both olive and mustard oil have strong scents and may thus be distracting rather than relaxing for some clients. Mustard oil can also be a skin irritant.

Which scalp conditions benefit from the use of oils?

- ***Alopecia***

This is sudden and severe hair loss, usually caused by stress, shock, illness, chemotherapy and sometimes pregnancy. It is temporary and should not be confused with male pattern baldness, when hair loss is permanent. The bald patches are random and sometimes become red and/or scaly. An oil massage helps the client to relax, which can lessen the effect of the problem, conditions the scalp and stimulates hair growth. Clients should be encouraged to massage their scalp at home between treatments.

- ***Dandruff (pityriasis capitis/simplex)***

Dandruff is a very common condition. It causes scales of dry skin to rub off the scalp into the hair. Often it can be treated with a shampoo. However, in more severe cases an oil massage will help by conditioning and reducing the dryness of the scalp.

- ***Eczema***

Eczema causes the scalp to become dry, itchy, scaly and red. In some cases the scaly areas bleed. Oil massage can help twofold: since an attack of eczema is often caused by stress, the relaxing effects of the treatment can help reduce its recurrence; the oils used will help condition the scalp and reduce the itchiness. Olive oil is particularly good at treating eczema, but mustard oil should never be used.

Common ailments that would benefit from Indian Head Massage include:

- Bell's Palsy
- headache
- temporo-mandibular joint tension (TMJ syndrome)
- tinnitus
- sycosis barbae (Barber's Itch)

You now know the techniques and benefits of Indian head massage. The next section explains the practicalities of carrying out a treatment.

CARRYING OUT A TREATMENT

One of the major practical benefits of Indian head massage is that it does not require the client to undress. This is very useful for two reasons: first, the nervous client or the client who is having a massage for the first time may feel uncomfortable about undressing and will feel reassured if this is not needed; second, the therapist needs very little equipment and can dispense with the changing facilities, towels or couch required for full body massage which means it is possible to work in a variety of environments, including the workplace.

What equipment is required?

The height of the client will affect the therapist's ability to reach their head and neck and the therapist needs to take this into account in order to prevent damage to themselves. A height-adjustable chair with proper lumbar support is the best type because it supports the client and also prevents the therapist from stooping. If a height-adjustable chair is not used, the therapist will need to use some form of bolster or cushion to adjust the client's height accordingly. If using oils for the scalp, a towel should be placed over the shoulders and a selection of base oils and, if required, essential oils should be easily accessible from the chair. (The same rule for all massages also applies to Indian head: keep at least one hand on the client once the treatment starts.)

What preparation is required for the client?

A consultation should be carried out to find out if there are any contraindications to Indian head massage. These are outlined in Chapter 4. However in addition note should be taken if the client has any of the following:

- pediculosis (lice)
- any contagious scalp conditions
- migraine
- nerves
- osteoporosis
- encephalitis
- meningitis
- poliomyelitis.

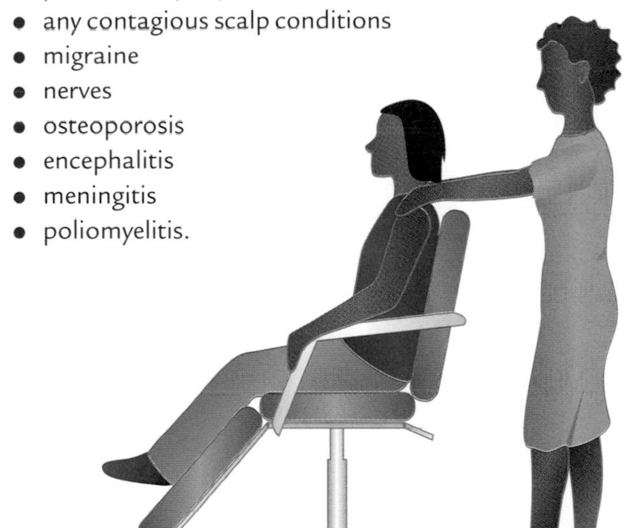

Carrying out treatment

Clients should remove all obstacles to treatment such as jewellery, glasses and hair accessories and should be advised to wear something light through which it is possible to massage the shoulders and neck rather than thick jackets and jumpers. Long hair should be tied back until the scalp massage begins and then released. If necessary, hair should be brushed or combed to remove any products like hairspray, mousse, gel or wax.

What preparation is required for the therapist?

The therapist should be able to reach the shoulders, neck, face and head of the client without overstretching. Adjust the height of the chair if necessary. Low shoes should be worn and long hair tied back. The therapist's posture and self-care is very important:

- keep back and legs straight but not rigid; the knees should be soft not locked
- adjust the position of the feet from standing to striding (see pp 60–61) when more pressure is needed
- relax the shoulders and upper back and avoid rolling shoulders up to the ears
- keep the head and neck aligned; avoid hanging the head and thus putting pressure on the neck and spine; lower the eyes rather than the whole head to look down and try to position the client so that it is not necessary to look down throughout the treatment
- keep the wrists straight and try to vary the movements to prevent repetitive strain injuries
- exercise the hands and wrists regularly
- keep hands scrupulously clean especially if using oils.

After treatment

Offer the client a glass of water and allow them a few minutes to 'wake up' from the deep relaxation. Explain that they may experience various reactions to treatment and that there is nothing to worry about. The body has been stimulated and relaxed and it is now adjusting to this by ridding itself of toxins and working on any problem areas that have been treated. Common reactions include:

- increased desire to urinate
- intensified emotional reactions
- tiredness
- lightheadedness
- aching muscles
- increase in production of mucous from the nasal passages
- healing crisis where symptoms become worse for a few hours before they begin to improve.

You now know what Indian head Massage is, what it does, which techniques are required and how to carry out a treatment.

11 Other complementary therapies

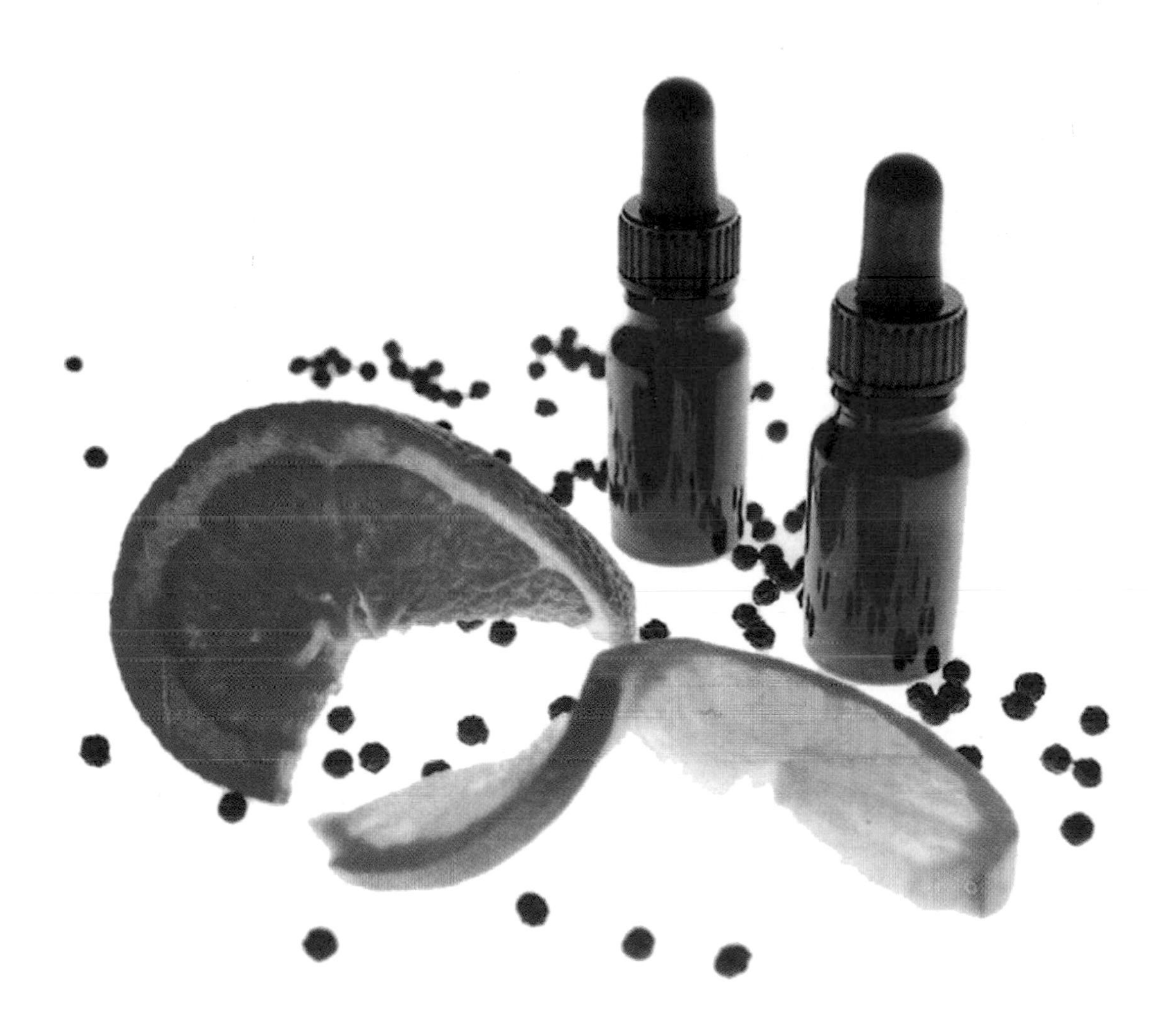

In Brief

Massage is only one of many complementary and holistic therapies. This chapter gives a brief overview of others. Some massage therapists combine therapies in treatments. For example aromatherapy and acupressure are both compatible with massage treatments.

Learning objectives

The target knowledge of this chapter is:

- **the definition of other complementary therapies.**

Acupressure

Acupressure is the same as acupunture but with the use of thumb or knuckles rather than needles. Pressure is applied along meridians to release the body's own energy – chi – to help relieve pain and encourage the body to heal itself . The massage is similar to Shiatsu, but performed directly onto the skin with the use of a light oil or talc.

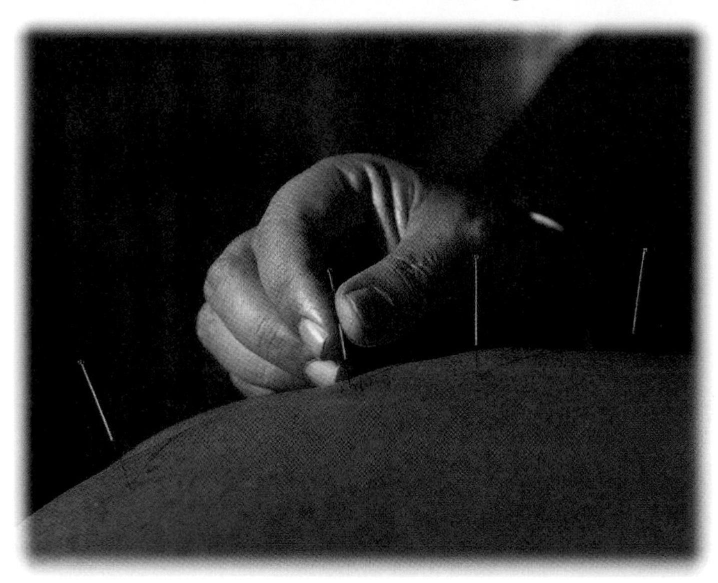

Acupuncture

An ancient Chinese therapy, now being used increasingly in the West, acupuncture is the insertion of very fine needles into the skin at certain points to help relieve pain and improve the body's own healing mechanisms. The points are on meridians (energy channels). If there is a blockage in energy then a part of the body connected to that meridian may become ill or weak. The needles are thought to release the blockage and help the body to heal itself.

Alexander technique

The Alexander technique encourages healing and better health through better posture and awareness of how the body is used. It is especially useful for backache and headaches. It was developed by an actor called Frederick

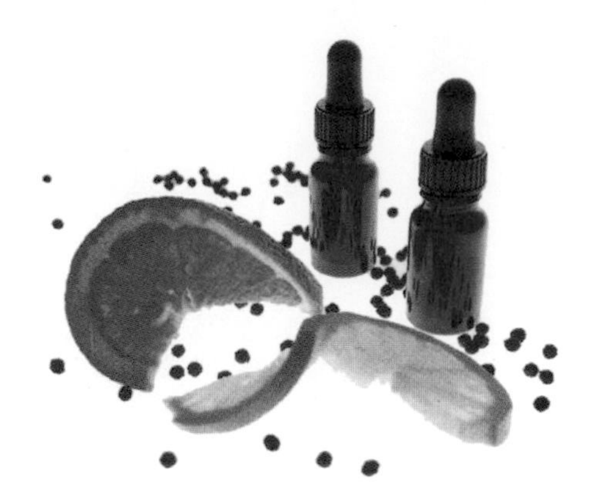

Mathias Alexander who discovered that improving his posture stopped him losing his voice.

Bach flower remedies

Dr Edward Bach, a doctor and a practising homeopath, turned away from both traditional medicine and homeopathy believing that there was a more natural and holistic way to treat illness. He developed these thirty-eight remedies, which are infusions of plants with water and alcohol, based on his research in the countryside. The remedies aim to treat mental and emotional problems, which often precede and cause physical symptoms.

Bowen technique

The Bowen technique, developed in Australia by Thomas A. Bowen, aims to rebalance the body holistically using gentle moves on tissues. A Bowen practitioner can feel whether muscles are stressed or tense and use the moves to release this build-up. The light rolling movements stimulate the body's energy flows. It is not a massage or a manipulation but a gentle process that encourages the body to heal itself.

Chiropractic

A chiropractor manipulates the joints of the body, specifically the spine, in order to relieve pain. It works on the basis that pain is often caused by a nerve which is not functioning properly and thus the spine, through which the central nervous

system runs, is the focus of the therapy. It is especially useful for lower back and neck pain as well as headaches.

Herbalism

Herbalism is the use of plants, usually the whole plant, to make herbal remedies. It is an ancient, traditional medicine – what is now considered 'traditional medicine' only replaced it in the last three hundred years.

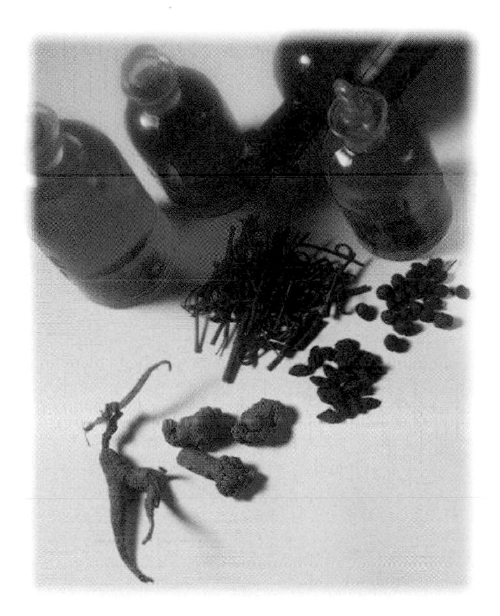

Homeopathy

Homeopathy treats like with like. By using minute doses of the bacteria, virus or substance which has caused the problem in the first place (i.e. cat hair in a remedy for an allergy to cat hairs) the treatment builds up the patient's resistance and immunity to the problem, substance or bacteria. Many homeopathic remedies have to be used and even stored well away from strong smells because such smells can reduce their effectiveness.

Iridology

By studying the irises (the coloured parts of the eyes) of a patient and noting any changes, iridologists can diagnose physical and psychological problems.

Kinesiology

Kinesiology is an holistic treatment that focuses on testing the muscles and energy meridians to discover and then treat the body's imbalances on all levels: chemically, energetically, physically and mentally. Using different positions and the application of pressure to the limbs, the kinesiologist can determine whether there are any energy blocks in the body and correct them through firm massage. Kinesiology is preventative and, like many complementary therapies, aims to treat the whole person.

Osteopathy

Like a chiropractor, an osteopath manipulates the joints of the body. Osteopaths work on the basis that the body's structure and function are interdependent: if the structure is damaged in any way it will affect the function. By manipulating joints and bones they can correct structural problems which will improve the body's function.

Physiotherapy

Physiotherapy uses physical exercises, massage and the application of pressure to relieve physical pain and muscular tension. It is often used to re-educate the body in cases of major surgery, illness, or an accident.

Reiki/spiritual healing

Reiki means universal life force energy in Japanese. Reiki healers act as channels for this universal energy to pass into the patient. By using hands in certain positions on different parts of the body, the healer is said to draw energy to the body, promoting healing, balance and relaxation.

Reflexology

This holistic therapy treats the whole person, particularly weak or ill areas, by using the feet as 'maps' of the body. On

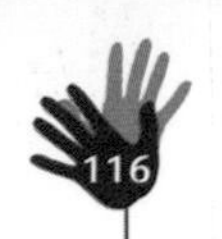

the feet there are points or zones which correspond to organs and systems of the body. By pressing on one of these points, the corresponding organ in the body is affected. For example, pressing on the tip of the big toe will cause a response in the brain and, vice versa, if there is a problem with the brain the reflexologist will recognise the symptoms of this in the big toe. This relationship, between a point on the foot and another part of the body is known as a reflex. A trained reflexologist uses finger or thumb pressure on each of the zones to find the problem areas. He or she then applies more pressure which helps the corresponding part of the body to heal. Some professionals use reflexology techniques during massage treatment.

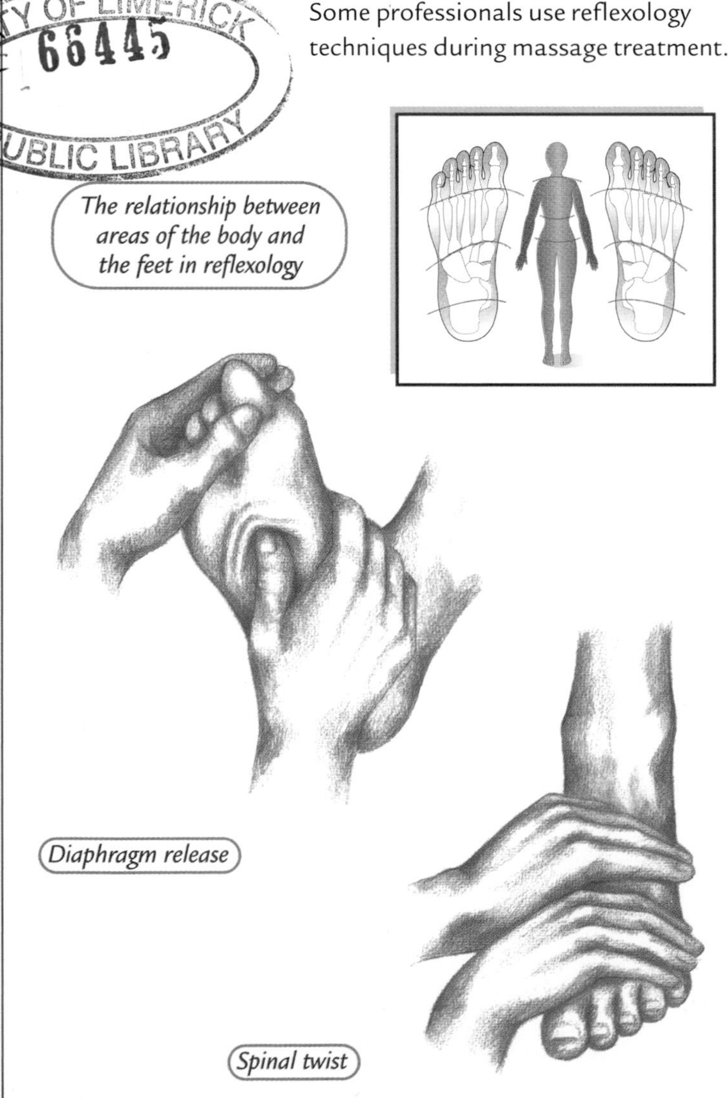

The relationship between areas of the body and the feet in reflexology

Diaphragm release

Spinal twist

Shiatsu

Shiatsu is a form of acupressure: the use of finger or thumb pressure on points along meridians (energy channels) to help relieve pain and encourage the body to heal itself. The pressure points are the same as those used in acupuncture. It is performed with the client clothed.

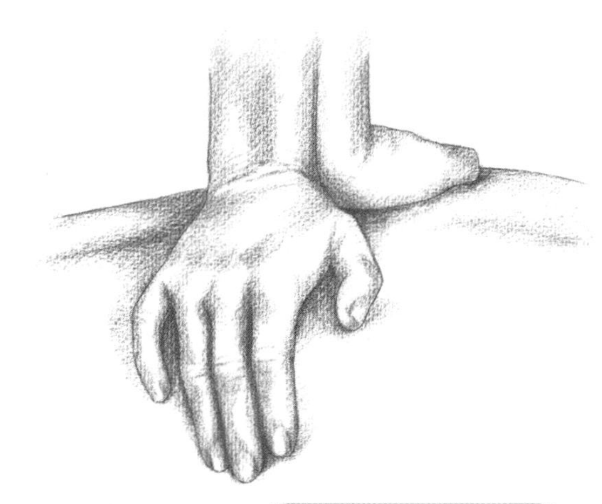

Shiatsu – using the heel of the hand to give a more general stimulation

Yoga/Meditation

Both yoga and meditation have long been known to have beneficial, holistic effects and they are very useful self-help therapies. They teach the learner to have control of the body and mind. Yoga does this through physical exercise, including adopting different postures, relaxation techniques and breathing exercises. Meditation uses different focuses (such as visualisation, a candle or a mantra) to help a person find calm and a sense of their own centre. Meditation has the physiological effects of a short sleep, i.e. the body goes into the healing and recharging mode it adopts when we sleep, allowing the muscles to relax and the circulation to become more efficient.

You now know details of several other complementary therapies.

Bibliography

- Beck, Mark, *The Theory and Practice of Therapeutic Massage*, Tarrytown, NY: Milady, 1988.
- Maxwell-Hudson, Claire, *The Complete Book of Massage*, London: Dorling Kindersley, 1988.
- McGuinness, Helen, *Holistic Therapies*, London: Hodder and Stoughton, 2000.
- McGuinness, Helen, *Indian Head Massage: Therapy Basics*, London: Hodder and Stoughton, 2000.
- Mitchell, Stewart, *Massage: a Practical Introduction*, Shaftesbury: Element, 1992.
- Tucker, Louise, *An Introductory Guide to Anatomy and Physiology*, revised edition, Cambridge: Holistic Therapy Books, 2000.
- Tucker, Louise, *An Introductory Guide to Aromatherapy*, Cambridge: Holistic Therapy Books, 2000.
- Wittlinger, H. and G., *Introduction to Dr. Vodder's Manual Lymph Drainage*, 2nd revised edition, Vol. 1: basic Karl F Haug Publishers. Heildelberg

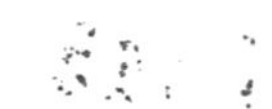

Glossary

Active movement: movement which requires client's participation

Acupressure : ancient Chinese therapy using thumb or finger pressure at acupoints along energy meridians in the body to unblock energy

Acupuncture: ancient Chinese therapy using needles inserted at acupoints along energy meridians in the body to unblock energy

Adenosine Triphosphate (ATP): a high energy phosphate molecule required to provide energy for cellular function

After care advice: advice given after a treatment to help maintain the effects of the treatment and the possible reactions that could occur

Allopathic: traditional Western medicine

Alexander technique: encourages healing and better health through improved posture and awareness of how the body is used

Amma: Ancient Chinese massage relying on treating specific points on the body

Aromatherapy: the use of essential oils for relaxation and the improvement of physical and emotional well-being

Ayurvedic medicine: The Ayurveda (from Sanskrit, *ayur* meaning 'life' and *veda*

'knowledge') is an ancient medical text about the arts of healing and prolonging life and it still forms the basis of much medical knowledge in India today.

Bach flower remedies: an infusion of plants with water and alcohol to treat mental and emotional problems

Blood pressure: the force that the blood exerts on the walls of the blood vessels as transmitted from the heart

Bowen technique: rebalancing the body holistically using gentle moves on tissues

Carbohydrates: are the body's energy providers

Carrier oil: neutral vegetable oil used in a blend with essential oil as a massage medium

Cellulite: a type of fat, mainly affecting women, causing dimpling and puckering of the skin. The formation of cellulite is linked to the hormones oestrogen and progesterone

Champissage: a percussion massage movement using both hands together in a 'prayer' position in a rhythmic movement

Chiropractic: manipulating the joints of the body, especially the spine, to relieve pain

Compression: the application of pressure to the body using the heel of the hand or fist to push the muscle tissue against the bone

Connective Tissue Massage (CTM): a form of stretching to release the fluids trapped within the connective tissue between the muscle fibres

Consultation: discussion with client to find out their needs and requirements and to find out any contraindications

Contraindication: reason why treatment cannot take place

Deep: below the surface; area furthest from skin

Desquamation: Natural shedding of skin cells

Effleurage: a gentle, relaxing stroke generally used at the beginning and end of a massage sequence or work on one particular section

Essential fatty acids: fats that cannot be produced by the body so must be supplied by the diet. These are Omega 3 and Omega 6

Essential oil: an aromatic, volatile substance extracted from plant material, with tiny molecules making it easy to be absorbed by the skin

Fats: an essential nutrient that provides energy, energy storage, and insulation and contour to the body

Friction: firm, rubbing technique which pushes layers of tissue against each other in order to stretch muscle fibres and release tension. Used as focus on specific area of body.

Galen: Greek who worked for the Roman Emperor, wrote many medical books stressing the use of massage for health purposes.

Herbalism: the use of plants to make herbal remedies

Herodicus: fifth-century physician and teacher of Hippocrates, wrote about the benefits of massage

Hippocrates: known as the father of medicine, believed all doctors needed to know how to use massage for healing purposes. Hippocrates called it anatripsis – 'the art of rubbing a part upward, not downward'

Holistic massage: a form of Swedish massage which takes into account not only the whole body including the mind and spirit

Homeopathy: treats like with like to build up the patient's resistance and immunity

Hypertonic drinks: a highly concentrated drink containing more sugar particles and electrolytes than the body's own fluids resulting in slower absorption than water

Hypotonic drinks: weak solution containing fewer particles of sugar and electrolytes than the body's own fluids resulting in faster absorption into the body than water

Indian Head Massage: uses and adapts classic Swedish massage techniques for treating the scalp, face, neck, shoulders and upper arms

Insertion of muscle: the moving end of a muscle; the muscle always works by moving away from its insertion, towards the origin

Integral biology: the study of our environment's effect on our physical and mental health

Iridology: physical and psychological problems seen in changes in the iris of the eye

Isotonic drinks: approximately the same number of particles in water as body fluids resulting in absorption into the body as quickly, if not quicker than water

Kinesiology: testing of the muscles and energy meridians to discover and treat the body's imbalances

Lactic acid: by-product of oxygen deficiency in muscles; if muscle is tired and running out of oxygen but continues to be used (e.g. when an athlete over-exercises) then lactic acid builds up causing a burning pain and stiffness. The muscle needs to rest in order to allow a fresh supply of oxygen to reach it and the lactic acid to be removed.

Ling, Per Henrik (1776-1839): a physiologist and fencing master. He was from Sweden and massage is still referred to as Swedish massage because of his influence. In the eighteenth and nineteenth centuries he developed a system of movements which he found helpful for improving his health and maintaining his physical condition. These movements are known as the Ling System.

Local: refers to a particular area or effect as opposed to whole body

Lymphatic drainage massage: is a system of techniques that help the lymphatic system function effectively

Massage: use of hands or mechanical means to manipulate soft tissues of body

Medium: substance used to aid massage movements. Talc, oil, gel, cream and anti-inflammatory rubs can be used.

Muscle Energy technique (MET): a variety of techniques that involve restricted or resistive movements to stretch muscles

Muscle tone: the degree of contraction of muscle fibres; at any one time there are always some muscle fibres contracting and this gives the body its normal shape and posture

Neuromuscular technique (NMT): a form of friction movement holding thumb or finger over a sore point and increasing pressure gradually to the limit of the client's pain threshold

Oedema: swelling of tissue through increase of its interstitial fluid volume

Origin of muscle: the fixed end of a muscle; the muscle always works towards its origin

Osteopathy: manipulating the joints and bones to correct structural problems which will improve the body's functions

Palpation: feeling muscles to assess damage and how to treat it

Passive movement: movement which requires no client involvement

Percussion: stimulating stroke using repetitive, brisk movements which 'wake up', tone and energise the body

Petrissage: compression stroke used to manipulate tissues and muscles. Resembles kneading; helps to break down tension.

Physiotherapy: the use of physical exercises, massage and the application of pressure to relieve physical pain and muscular tension

Pressure points: points along the energy meridians

Pressure techniques: those that require application of pressure, usually from palm or heel of hand, fist, fingers or thumbs

Proteins: necessary for the growth and formation of new tissues, and also for repairing damaged tissues

Record card: an information sheet with all the client's personal details on and the treatments given

Referral area: area associated with another area of the body used in treatment when one area cannot be touched; e.g. if knee is damaged the knee' referral area, the elbow, can be treated instead

Reflexology: specialised foot massage treating the whole person by using the feet as 'maps' of the body. There are points or zones that correspond to organs and systems of the body. By pressing on one of these points, the corresponding organ in the body is affected

Reiki/spiritual healing: the use of the healer's hands on different parts of the body to draw energy to the patient's body promoting healing, balance and relaxation

Shiatsu: system of applying pressure to certain points on the body to improve circulation and health. It is performed with the client clothed.

Soft Tissue Release (STR): combination of pressure and movement causing the muscle fibres to lengthen and stretch

Stress: is any factor that threatens our physical or mental well-being. There are two types of stress: positive which can help some people perform to the best of their abilities, negative is any factor causing us to respond by worrying, panicking or losing our concentration.

Superficial: surface of body; area closest to skin

Swedish massage: system of massage movements developed by and named after Swedish physiologist Per Henrik Ling. Movements were called effleurage, petrissage and percussion.

Tabla: superficial tapping movement using the tops of the fingers or the heels of the hands

Toxin: substance that can harm or damage the body if not removed; may be ingested or a by-product of body's functioning

Tsubo: Japanese name for the points of the body used in massage (based on Ancient Chinese practice)

Vibration: manual or mechanical method of moving flesh with gentle vibrations; can be stimulating or relaxing.

Waste: substances produced by body's functions which need to be removed in order for body to continue working effectively, e.g. carbon dioxide, urea

Working position: stance used by therapist to carry out treatment

Yoga: teaches the learner to have control over the mind and body through physical exercise.

Index

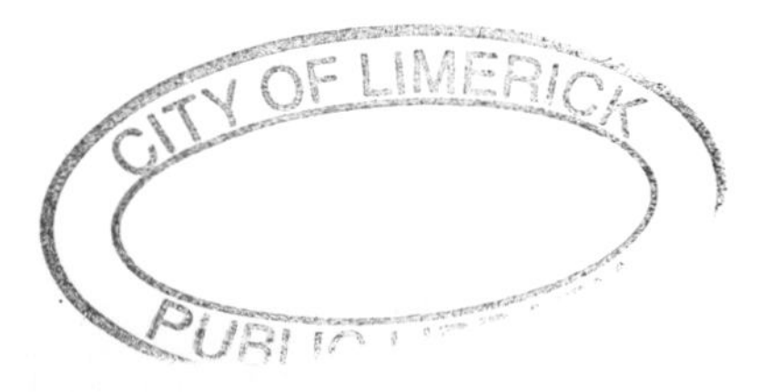